What  Didn't Tell You About

Childhood Constipation

By

Wendy Hayden

WHAT YOUR DOCTOR DIDN'T TELL YOU ABOUT CHILDHOOD CONSTIPATION

First edition. July 5, 2019.

Written by Wendy Hayden.

Introduction

My son's struggle with chronic constipation, and the side effects he experienced from Miralax, inspired me to learn everything I could as a parent to help my son. I began to research natural ways to combat constipation after my son developed horrible side effects from Miralax, which had been prescribed by his pediatric gastroenterologist.

I found that there were many parents whose children were also experiencing significant side effects from Miralax and many more who wanted to avoid using a chemical laxatives.

Over the next few years, I started my website www.NaturalConstipationSolutions.com and multiple Facebook groups and now I've written this book, to share what I have learned to help other families, like yours. I have been lucky enough to help thousands of families get their child off of Miralax, or avoid Miralax, find the reason why their child became constipated in the first place and get a game plan to help end their child's chronic constipation.

I am not a doctor or a medical professional. I am just a mom who has been through the struggle of trying to help my son with his chronic constipation. I hope my experience can help you with your child.

My youngest son struggled with constipation from birth and was diagnosed with reflux as an infant. He had terrible gas, his stool smelled like it was rotting and he was in pain when he would pass a bowel movement.

I exclusively breastfed him, avoided milk and cruciferous veggies in my diet trying to help him. I always considered myself a pretty "crunchy" mama and tried so hard to feed my son a healthy diet and help him with his constipation naturally. When he started to eat solids, his constipation and gas got worse. He was dairy free from birth, I bought as much organic foods as I could afford and I tried to feed him healthy foods but he was still struggling.

When my son was 16 months old, he contracted Salmonella. He was hospitalized and put on Intravenous antibiotics for 5 days. The antibiotics saved his life but damaged his gut. His constipation worsened, he slipped from the 80th percentile in weight, down to the 10th percentile and wasn't growing. I took him to multiple doctors trying to figure out what was wrong with him and what I could do to help him. He was in so much pain and would scream from his belly hurting. He was anemic but when his pediatrician prescribed iron for his anemia, it worsened his constipation and caused even more gut pain.

At 18 months, he was diagnosed with IgA deficiency and gluten intolerance, suspected celiac disease. I immediately put him on a gluten free diet and he started to do a little better. This was over 10 years ago and it was much harder to find gluten free options. It took months for me to figure out how to do a gluten free diet for him as gluten is hidden in many places that aren't obvious. As I got better at feeding him gluten free, he improved but something still wasn't right.

I took him to his pediatrician and just about every pediatric gastroenterologist in my city. Eventually, we were referred a university hospital about 2 hours from my home. We made an appointment with the head of Pediatric Gastroenterology.

The Gastroenterologist asked me questions, read his records and took an X-ray. The X-ray showed that my son was full of stool. Even though he had been having a daily bowel movement, he was completely backed up. What my son was passing was soft stool that was leaking around the backed up stool.

The Gastro diagnosed my son with genetic Megacolon, a birth defect where the nerves did not travel down his colon properly during the first trimester. This caused my son to have a lack of feeling when he needed to go and a lack of ability to push out the stool. Because of this, stool had backed up in his intestines and stretched them out, making it even harder for him to pass a normal bowel movement.

The Gastro prescribed a Miralax clean out to flush out his intestines. I was to give my 4 year old son two capfuls of Miralax a day for 3 days and then I was told by the doctor to give him a 1/2 cap of Miralax a day indefinitely after the initial clean out. The doctor told me that because of his Megacolon, he would need to be on Miralax for life. I questioned the safety and the doctor told me that it was "an inert sugar" and "completely safe for long-term use." "Safe as water" is a phrase he used. Since the doctor was very well-respected and head of his department at a university teaching hospital, I trusted him.

Shortly after, my son was given 4X's the daily dose by a family member in confusion over the clean out dose versus the daily dose. My older son had Rotavirus at the time and my youngest son ended up catching the Rotavirus on top of the clean-out dose. He ended up in the hospital again, this time for 4 days. He was diagnosed with dehydration and Rotavirus and needed to be put on IVs and antibiotics again.

My son was on a 1/2 cap of Miralax a day for about a year and a half. Over time, he started to tic, he had gut pain that would double him over prior to having a bowel movement and he developed massive anxiety to the point where he had to be with me wherever I went. He went as far as sitting on the bath mat when I showered because he would panic if I was out of sight. He was having trouble potty training, he was obsessively lining his toys up and spinning in circles.

It was a slow and gradual increase in these behaviors so it wasn't obvious what was causing them. Then, after a round of antibiotics for a suspected parasite, these behaviors escalated quickly and were really scary. His doctor got him into the local children's hospital for an emergency evaluation with a neurologist.

His doctor suspected PANS (Pediatric Acute-onset Neuropsychiatric Syndrome) or PANDAS (Pediatric Autoimmune Neuropsychiatric Disorders associated with streptococcal infections) but my son hadn't had strep or any other triggers that we could think of. We had a psychiatric evaluation done and I was told that Tourette's plus OCD and anxiety were suspected. They referred us to an Occupational Therapist who also diagnosed him with Sensory Processing Disorder and low tone and he began twice weekly Occupational Therapy.

My son was still having pain before bowel movements and, even though all of the doctors had assured me that it wasn't connected to Miralax, I thought it was. I started to wean him off of Miralax and found a new Integrative doctor. The new doctor told me that we needed to get my son off of Miralax asap and keep him off. He said to use Magnesium to help with constipation while we healed his gut, put him on an organic whole food diet, and to work on healing his gut with bone broth, fermented foods and drinks and supplements.

My son was doing really well on magnesium and his tics, anxiety, and OCD were improving over the next few months. Then, a family member gave him a dose of Miralax and the behaviors and tics all came back, even worse than when he was on Miralax the first time around. Furthermore, he had hallucinations, slurred speech, panic attacks, skin picking, anxiety, night terrors, tics, etc. It took months to get him back to where he was before this Miralax exposure. It became very clear that Miralax was causing the mental health issues that my son was having.

My son has been off of Miralax for years. My son's tics are much better and only flare up when he is stressed or comes in contact with a product with PEG (Polyethylene Glycol, the only ingredient in Miralax) in it.

Healing his gut and repopulating his gut flora has helped his bowel movements to be very regular, his anxiety improved, and his sensory behaviors are much better that he had while on Miralax. It has been a long road and I don't know what the long-term ramifications will be from Miralax use for my son, but thankfully he is continuing to do better over time.

Ideally, you would be able to get help with your child's chronic constipation from their pediatrician or pediatric gastroenterologist. But in my experience personally, and with the thousands of parents I have worked with in the Facebook groups I have been involved with, most doctors just tell you to use Miralax or another laxative and send you on your way.

If you can, I highly recommend working with a Functional Medicine Doctor or Integrative Medical Doctor. They are trained to get to the root cause of the problem instead of just prescribing a medication for the symptom. Constipation is a symptom of a bigger problem or combination of problems. When you work on resolving the problems that are causing the constipation, the constipation will resolve.

Unfortunately, not everyone has access to these doctors. Either because there aren't any near you or because you can't afford to take your child to one. Many do not take insurance because they spend a significant amount of time with each patient's case, going over medical records and then with the patient in person. My son's doctor spends an hour with us at each appointment. A regular doctor is not able to spend that amount of time with each patient. A

Functional or Integrative doctor is worth every cent, but I also realize that the cost is prohibitive to many families.

Beyond the fact that Miralax doesn't solve your child's constipation long term, it is also not approved by the FDA for use in children under 17 and not approved for use in anyone for longer than 7 days. At the time I am writing this, over 25,000 reports of adverse events have been reported to the FDA, some very serious including seizures and even deaths.

Unfortunately, many doctors prescribe it to young children and even infants. One of my readers told me that her baby was a 32 week premie who struggled with constipation from birth. When her baby was 4 weeks old, the doctor prescribed Miralax. The baby wouldn't have even been out of the womb yet and was being given a toxic drug.

Many parents have reached out telling their stories of their child being put on Miralax and other laxatives for years with no resolution of their child's constipation and in many cases, the constipation worsening over time. Instead of getting to the cause of the constipation, their doctors just upped the dose of the laxative. Many times, these children began experiencing behavior issues, mental health issues and some were even suicidal.

These heartbreaking stories, along with my son's struggle, convinced me that this book was necessary to give dedicated parents an alternative to giving their child laxatives for years.

I am not a doctor or other medical professional. I am just a mom who has been through this struggle and came out the other side with a child who no longer has chronic constipation. I can't diagnose your child or give you medical advice. But, I can help you to figure out the questions to ask your doctor to get them to work with you on finding the root cause of your child's constipation.

It is exhausting to try to solve your child's chronic constipation on your own. But it is doable. You can find safe, natural treatments short term and also figure out why your child is constipated and solve their chronic constipation permanently.

On my website, I have a free bowel movement tracker you can download and print. The tracker will help you to track your child's bowel movements and the effectiveness of the interventions you will be trying.

https://naturalconstipationsolutions.com/bowel-movement-tracker/

Helping Your Child Have a Bowel Movement

Constipation in Infants

There isn't much that is more stressful than when your infant isn't feeling well. And when your baby is constipated, you are limited in what you can safely do to help them to poop. My son was constipated from birth. It was a constant struggle to get him to go regularly and to help him to not be in pain from gas and constipation.

Signs of constipation in infants include arching of their back when they go or before they go, crying when they have a bowel movement, the bowel movement being hard and difficult to pass, passing pebble shaped stool, straining, blood around their rectum or passing dark brown or green stools. On average babies 0-4 months of age poop 3-4 times a day. Once solids are introduced to their diet, some babies only poop once a day. Ideally, infants should be having a bowel movement after each time they eat although this can vary dramatically depending on their diet.

The first thing to look at with a constipated baby is, what is causing their constipation. If your baby has been constipated from birth, are they breastfed or formula fed? Did their constipation start when you introduced solid foods? Did their constipation begin when you weaned your baby? Thinking about this will give you clues to look at what you can do to help them.

Although some breastfed babies have a bowel movement after each feeding, it is also very common for breastfed babies not to have a bowel movement daily. Not going daily doesn't necessarily signal that they are constipated and need any interventions. But if they aren't going for 3 or 4 days or are in obvious pain or straining when they go, then it is time to try to figure out what is causing their constipation.

With breastfed babies, you need to look at **your** diet. Proteins from the food you eat will travel through your milk and into your baby. The most common culprits in constipation are dairy and gluten. Gluten is a protein commonly found in wheat, barley and triticale and some oats. They include pasta, bread, pizza, muffins etc. Other foods that can cause constipation in breastfed infants are foods like broccoli, onions, cauliflower, soy, and beans.

If you are nursing, doing an elimination diet will help you to find out what the culprits are causing issues for your baby. Eliminate gluten, diary, soy, beans, and cruciferous vegetables for 30 days. See if your babies symptoms improve. If they do, add one food type back in at a time. Wait at least 3-5 days in between reintroducing foods and see how your baby does.

Doing a food diary, where you write down what you eat and what your baby's bowel movements are like, can be super helpful in determining if something in your diet is causing their constipation.

It can be overwhelming to consider changing your diet and going dairy free and gluten free but it can make a huge difference in your child's gut health. The easiest and cheapest way to go gluten-free is to eat a whole food diet of meat, vegetables, and fruit, avoiding any processed foods and all bread, pasta, baked goods, and pizza. There are also so many excellent dairy and/or gluten-free products available now and most restaurants have gluten-free menus.

When looking at dairy-free substitutes, avoid any nondairy kinds of milk that contain carrageenan. Carrageenan can cause stomach distress. We'll go into more details on gluten and dairy in future chapters.

In addition to my son's constipation and rancid gas, gluten caused eczema. If your baby has eczema, that is a sign of a food intolerance or allergy and needs to be discussed with your baby's doctor. If the doctor just gives you hydrocortisone cream and sends you on your way, it is time to find a new doctor.

If your baby is formula fed, there are a few issues that can lead to constipation. Most formulas are iron fortified. Iron supplements and fortified formulas can cause constipation. Discuss other ways to get iron into your babies diet without using iron supplements such as diet. Iron rich foods such as chicken, fish and beef. Chicken liver is very high in iron. Eggs, molasses and spinach are also good sources of iron. If you are nursing, increasing iron in your diet can help.

Some babies do well on an organic formula that is formulated for sensitive digestive systems. Just switching to an organic formula might help your baby. Organic formulas do not have any GMO ingredients and do not use toxic weed killers and pesticides on the feed the cows eat.

Nutramigen and Alimentum are formulas that are extensively hydrolyzed. They break the casein, a cow's milk protein, into pieces that are more digestible for some infants. Neocate and Ele-Care are hypoallergenic formula options. They are amino acid-based or elemental formulas. If other options don't work for your baby, these are ones to try. There are also prescription formulas that you can discuss with your pediatrician. Insurance will often cover prescription formulas which can be helpful because they are very expensive.

I would also ask your physician to run tests to see if your infant is allergic to cow's milk, if so, and the amino acid-based formulas are still constipating your baby, then a goat's milk-based formula can be a really good option for your baby. My son had green stools when he got dairy so if your baby has green stools, I would ask your pediatrician to test for a cow's milk allergy or intolerance.

If your baby is intolerant to cow's milk, then most cow's milk formulas can cause constipation. Many people substitute soy formula instead of cow's milk but I do not recommend soy formula. Soy, unless it is organic, is genetically modified. Many babies react to it. Soy is also a known endocrine disruptor and can cause hormone issues down the road including precocious puberty in boys and girls. Soy is also constipating for many children. I would avoid all soy formulas.

You can also discuss with your pediatrician or research yourself whether there is a milk bank in your area where you can get donated breast milk.

If a change in the formula for a formula-fed infant or a change in your diet for a breastfed infant doesn't help with constipation then there are other things that need to be examined to determine what the root cause of your child's constipation is.

If your baby has started solids, and that is when their constipation started, then an elimination diet for your baby is in order. If your baby is under a year old, they are getting the nutrition they need from breastmilk or formula. Any foods they eat, are fun, help them to learn to eat, and are tasty, but they aren't necessary. You aren't going to starve your baby by going back a step or two in solid foods.

Grains, veggies or even fruit can cause constipation. My son couldn't tolerate many fruits that are recommended for helping with constipation. He would get horrible gas and would be in pain after eating them. He needed to do a low fructose diet to help with gas and constipation.

To do an elimination diet for your baby, remove gluten, dairy, and cruciferous veggies for 30 days and then add them back one at a time to see what is causing your infants constipation. Other foods can cause constipation but these are the most common. I highly recommend starting a food diary and note what your baby is eating and what their bowel movements are like every day. This can help you to track what food is causing a problem.

Baby cereals are often very constipating, especially if they are iron fortified. One wonderful first food that you can offer your baby is homemade bone broth. It is simple and inexpensive to make. I recommend using bones from organic, grass-fed animals for your bone broth, add in lots of organic veggies and they will get the benefit of the nutrients plus the collagen in the bones which will help heal their gut.

Avoiding grain-based baby foods like cereals, cookies, teething biscuits, crackers etc can help with your babies constipation. For babies that are ready for fruit, organic prune purees can help. Some families have success with a quinoa cereal, instead of using rice cereal or oatmeal.

When introducing foods to your baby, only introduce one food at a time for a few days to make sure that your infant doesn't have a reaction to it before adding another food.

Low tone can also be a root cause of constipation in children. If your baby was late to turn over or has an unusual crawl like an army crawl or they sit upright and pull themselves along on their bottom, then Low Tone/Hypotonia is something to look into.

Your pediatrician should be able to give you an idea if this is an issue for your baby and if he or she suspects that it is, they will refer you to an occupational therapist, who will do an evaluation on your baby to see if your child has hypotonia. We will go into more detail on low tone in a future chapter.

If you or your baby's other parent or grandparents have had constipation issues, have been diagnosed with celiac, IBS, food allergies or intolerances or thyroid problems, then getting your baby tested for these things is critical because many times these issues are genetic.

While you are working on finding the root cause of their constipation, there are some safe things that you can do to help your infant have comfortable bowel movements.

Add a full spectrum mineral supplement that is safe for infants to your baby's diet. Omniblue Ocean Minerals is one such supplement and is safe for infants. Omniblue has magnesium, which helps constipation by relaxing the muscles in the intestines and also by attracting water to increase the water in the colon. This makes the stool softer and easier to pass. Add a drop or two to your infant's formula at each feeding. Omniblue has a very strong flavor and must be diluted.

If you are breastfeeding, you can pump a small amount of milk and add the minerals to the milk or mix with a small amount of water and syringe into your baby's mouth. You will need to experiment to find the correct dose on minerals that your infant needs to have soft, easy to pass stools without getting stools that are too loose.

If your child is having a lot of gas, organic gripe water can really help, and is safe for infants. I would not use simethicone drops.

My son had horrible gas as an infant. His bowel movements and gas smelled like something was rotting. When I would change his diaper the smell would be so bad that you could smell it at the other end of our house. I was breastfeeding him and had eliminated dairy, soy, and cruciferous veggies out of my diet trying to figure out what was causing his painful, rancid smelling gas. Gripe water really helped but I knew that was just a bandaid on his problem and wasn't solving it long term.

My son ended up getting diagnosed with celiac at 18 months after he had IgA testing. If your child is having similar issues, ask your doctor to test for celiac disease.

Doing a tummy massage can help your infant to have a bowel movement. There are many ways to do massage on a constipated infant. One way is to lay the flat of your hand on your baby's navel (as long as the cord has fallen off and is healed) and do small, increasingly larger circles around their tummies with gentle pressure. Another option is to start under their rib cage, and with gentle pressure, stroke down their belly. Bicycling your baby's legs and pushing their legs up into their tummy is also very effective for releasing gas and getting things moving.

Infant sized glycerine suppositories or infant enemas are one way to get things moving if your baby has hard stool low down in his or her rectum. If you see your baby pushing and nothing is coming out, or only hard balls are coming out, these can help to lubricate the stool and anus and make it easier for your baby to push the poop out. You can also lubricate the anus with organic coconut oil to make it easier for the hard stool to come out without causing damage.

An Epsom salt bath can help relax your baby, replenish magnesium stores and help him or her to have a bowel movement. Just a warning, sometimes the bowel movement will happen in the bath! For an infant, add 1/2 cup of Epsom salt to the bath water. If you have chlorinated water, add 1/4 cup of baking soda as well. Let your baby play or soak in the water for at least 20 minutes. Epsom salt can be itchy when it dries on the skin so you may want to rinse your baby after their bath.

If your baby was born by c-section, he or she didn't get the benefit of your bacteria as they came through the birth canal. Their first expo-sure to bacteria was hospital bacteria instead of their mother's. This can lead to constipation.

If your baby is formula fed, they aren't getting the beneficial bacteria that is in breastmilk. If your baby has been on antibiotics or if you have been on a lot of antibiotics before or during your pregnancy or while breastfeeding, then your baby may be lacking in the bacteria they need for proper digestion.

Supplementing with a high quality infant probiotic can make a huge improvement in your infant's constipation. Look for a probiotic made specifically for infants, ideally with multiple strains of bacteria. When supplementing with probiotics it is good to rotate through different ones to get the most variety of strains to avoid growing a monoculture of just a few strains of bacteria.

Taking your baby to a chiropractor might seem like an unusual thing to do for constipation but many parents have reported success in achieving bowel movements after having their infant adjusted. Look for a chiropractor who is experienced in adjusting infants. Unlike what you might expect, adjustments for infants are very gentle and can help with colic, constipation and sleep issues in infants. Many chiropractors also will help you with finding the root cause of your baby's constipation.

There are other serious problems that can cause constipation such as tethered cord, Hirchsprung's Disease, hypothyroidism, congenital megacolon, motility issues, tongue or lip tie. Ask your pediatrician to look into these issues if none of the above changes help.

If your pediatrician isn't helpful in figuring out why your baby is constipated and just recommends a laxative, it is time to try a new pediatrician. It is so important to handle constipation as early as possible. If your baby's doctor isn't on board with really helping you, then move on. Even if your pediatrician has been great with your older children, if they aren't helping you with this issue, you need a new doctor who will help you before your baby's constipation becomes entrenched.

Constipation in Toddlers

Toddlers can be willful and a challenge to parent on a good day, add in constipation and it is incredibly exhausting and frustrating.

They are independent enough to not want to do what you ask but not old enough to be able to discuss with them why they need to eat or drink something they don't like, or sit on the potty when they don't want to or make an effort to push out stool when it is uncomfortable. You can't reason with a toddler and you really can't reason with a constipated toddler!

Your child should be passing soft smooth sausage shaped stools about 1/2 the size of their wrist, 1-3 times a day. If your child is struggling to push out large, hard, bumpy stool, rabbit pellet type of stool or very soft liquid stool (this can be a sign of encopresis where the soft stool oozes around a blockage of hard stool further up the intestines) he or she is probably constipated.

If your child is having pee accidents along with constipation, the pee accidents are more than likely caused by the stool in the colon pushing on the bladder. Working on solving your child's constipation will often end pee accidents.

Many pediatricians and gastroenterologists prescribe Miralax for constipation. It dissolves in their drink and doesn't have much taste so it can be easy to get your child to take it. But Miralax hasn't been approved for use in children under 17 and hasn't been approved for use in anyone for more than 7 days. On top of that, as of the time I am writing this chapter, over 25,000 reports of adverse events related to Miralax have been reported to the FDA.

Some very serious adverse events include tics, rage, aggression, OCD, ADD, seizures, panic attacks, kidney problems, Autism-like behaviors, ODD, night terrors, learning delays, mouth sores, lack of growth, hallucinations, speech issues, numbness Issues, and number of pediatric deaths. Beyond the dangers of Miralax, it is just a bandaid on your toddler's constipation and won't solve the problem long term.

The first thing to look at with a constipated toddler is, what is causing their constipation?

If your toddler has been constipated from birth, were they breastfed or formula fed? Did their constipation start when you introduced solid foods? Did their constipation begin when you weaned them? Thinking about this will give you clues to look at what you can do to help them with their constipation.

It can be overwhelming to consider changing their diet, especially with toddlers who are notoriously picky, but it can make a huge difference in your child's gut health. Gluten and dairy are the most common causes of constipation. The easiest and cheapest way to go gluten-free is to eat a whole food diet of meat, vegetables, and fruit, avoiding any processed foods and all bread, pasta, baked goods, and pizza. There are also so many excellent dairy and/or gluten-free products available now and most restaurants have gluten-free menus. When looking at dairy-free substitutes, avoid any nondairy kinds of milk that contain carrageenan. Carrageenan can cause stomach distress.

I would also ask your physician to run tests to see if your toddler is allergic to cow's milk, if so, and the amino acid-based formulas are still constipating your toddler, then a goat's milk can be a really good option for your toddler. Toddlers do not need to be drinking any milk or formula at all. They are not reliant on milk or formula for nutrition like they are when they are babies.

Discontinuing all milk or formulas are an option if you can't find one that doesn't bother them. We'll go into more detail on dairy in a later chapter.

If your toddler's constipation started when you introduced solids, then an elimination diet is in order. Doing an elimination diet, where you go back to just one or two solid foods and gradually add other foods in, one at a time to see what is causing your toddler's constipation is a good place to begin. I highly recommend starting a food diary and note what your toddler is eating and what their bowel movements are like every day. This can help you to track what food might be causing a problem.

Baby cereals are often very constipating, especially if they are iron fortified. Iron supplements are very constipating.

One wonderful food that you can offer your toddler is homemade bone broth. It is simple and inexpensive to make. I recommend using bones from organic, grass-fed animals for your bone broth. Avoiding grain-based baby foods like cereals, cookies, teething biscuits, crackers etc can help with your toddler's constipation.

When introducing foods to your toddler, only introduce one food at a time and only give that food for a few days along with previous foods that haven't bothered him or her before introducing the next food to make sure that your toddler doesn't have a reaction to it before adding another food.

If a change in diet, doesn't help with constipation then there are other things that need to be examined to determine what the root cause of your child's constipation is.

Some possibilities to discuss with your pediatrician include tongue-tie, tethered spinal cord, Hirschsprung's disease, food allergies, motility issues, Celiac or gluten intolerance or hypothyroidism.

If you or your toddler's other parent or grandparents have had constipation issues, have been diagnosed with Celiac, IBS, Crohn's, food allergies or intolerances or thyroid problems, then getting your toddler tested for these things is critical.

Low tone can also be a root cause of constipation in children. If your toddler was late to turn over, crawl or walk or had an unusual crawl like an army crawl or they sat upright and pulled themselves along on their bottom, or sit in a W style instead of Chris/Cross/Applesauce style, then low tone or hypotonia is something to look into.

While you are working on finding the root cause of their constipation, there are some safe things that you can do to help your toddler have comfortable bowel movements.

Magnesium is very helpful with constipation. Magnesium works to help constipation by relaxing the muscles in the intestines and also by attracting water to increase the water in the colon. This makes the stool softer and easier to pass. Finding a full spectrum mineral supplement with magnesium is a good way to increase magnesium for your child.

Omniblue is a full spectrum mineral supplement that is safe for toddlers. Add a drop or two to your toddler's drink at each meal or mix in ketchup, dip, soup or applesauce. Omniblue has a very strong flavor and must be diluted. If you are breastfeeding you can pump a small amount of milk and add the minerals to the milk or mix with a small amount of water and syringe into your toddler's mouth. You will need to experiment to find the correct dose of minerals that your toddler needs to have soft, easy to pass stools without getting stools that are too loose. Use small frequent doses of magnesium to find out how much your child needs to have an ideal stool.

Doing a tummy massage can also help your toddler to have a bowel movement. There are many ways to do a tummy massage for constipation. You can start under your toddler's ribs with a flat hand and apply even pressure as you sweep their tummy down to their pubic bone, or you can start at their navel and with gentle pressure and a flat hand, slowly make circles, enlarging the circle with each pass.

Liquid glycerin suppositories are one way to get things moving if your toddler has hard stool low down in his or her rectum. If you see your toddler pushing and nothing is coming out or only hard balls are coming out, these can help to lubricate the stool and anus and make it easier for your toddler to push the poop out. You can also lubricate the anus with coconut oil to make it easier for the hard stool to come out without causing damage.

An Epsom salt bath can help relax your toddler, replenish magnesium stores and help him or her to have a bowel movement. Just a warning, sometimes the bowel movement will happen in the bath! For a toddler, I would recommend adding 1 cup of Epsom salt to the bath water. If you have chlorinated water, add 1/4 cup of baking soda as well. Let your toddler play or soak in the water around 20 minutes. Epsom salt can be itchy when it dries on the skin so you may want to rinse your toddler after.

If your baby was born by C-Section, he or she didn't get the benefit of your bacteria as they came through the birth canal. Their first exposure to bacteria was hospital bacteria instead of their mother's. This can lead to constipation.

If your toddler was formula fed, they aren't getting the beneficial bacteria that is in breastmilk. If your toddler has been on antibiotics or if you have been on a lot of antibiotics before or during your pregnancy, then your toddler may be lacking in the bacteria they need for proper digestion.

Supplementing with a probiotic can really make a huge improvement in your toddlers's constipation.

When supplementing with probiotics, it is good to rotate through different ones to get the most variety of strains to avoid growing a monoculture of just a few strains of bacteria.

Taking your toddler to a chiropractor might seem an unusual thing to do for constipation but many parents have reported a lot of success in achieving bowel movements after having their toddler adjusted. Look for a chiropractor who is experienced in adjusting children. Adjustments for toddlers are very gentle and can help with colic, constipation and sleep issues.

If your toddler's constipation started when you began working on potty training, your toddler is probably not ready mentally or physically to be potty trained yet. There is no magic age for when a child will be ready to potty train. Often children are ready between 2 and 3 years of age but some children aren't ready to potty train until well after they turn three, especially children who have struggled with constipation and have a fear of having a painful bowel movement.

One painful experience while sitting on the toilet can push back potty training for months, so it is best not to push a child to attempt to potty train until you have their constipation under control.

After you have them passing soft stools in their diapers regularly, then reintroduce potty training. Ideally your child will show interest in using the toilet and graduating out of their diaper or pull up before you attempt to get them to go on the toilet. This can prevent constipation from reoccurring when you work on potty training again. Going to the restroom when you or their other parent or grandparent or older siblings and modeling using the toilet, can help your toddler to feel more comfortable with attempting to go on the toilet.

I know that it can be frustrating when you are in a situation where your child needs to be potty trained for day care or pre-school and you are trying to get them ready for this big life step, but some children, especially ones who have struggled with chronic constipation, just may not be ready by the time the deadline rolls around.

I suggest talking with your child's pediatrician or pediatric gastro and seeing if you can get them to write you a letter for your child's day care or pre-school explaining why your child is delayed in potty training. Another option is to look into a home based day care or a pre-school co-op that is more flexible on potty training deadlines.

If your child has been constipated for a significant period of time, they may have lost the sensation of when they need to go because their colon and intestines can get stretched out and from nerve damage caused by chronic constipation or what is causing their chronic constipation. This makes potty training very difficult. Hirschprung's Disease and megacolon commonly cause problems for potty training because the child doesn't feel the urge to go.

Often, even if the child does not know that he or she needs to have a bowel movement, they often do give some signals when they are getting ready to have a bowel movement. Passing gas, exhibiting restlessness or anxiety, squatting down in a corner, getting very quiet, or hiding, can all be signs that a bowel movement is on it's way. If you notice these signs happening, then sitting your child on their potty or at least mentioning that you think they may need to try to go to the bathroom because you have noticed X, Y or Z behavior, behavior you feel is an indication that a bowel movement is coming, can help them to begin to recognize the signs of an impending bowel movement.

Instituting a "Try Time" 20-30 minutes after a meal and before bed or at any time they routinely have a bowel movement, can help to get your child to develop a routine of going. Keep the "Try Time" short, no more than 5-10 minutes, and relaxed. This is a good time to read to your child or let them have electronics, as long as the electronics aren't too distracting, so they can relax and try to go. If your child has any anxiety about "Try Time" and resists, then go back to diapers or pull ups and try again down the road when they shows signs of being ready to potty train.

Some signs of being ready for potty training are as follows: telling you when they have gone in their pull up and need to be changed, pulling at their dirty diaper or acting irritated by it, hiding when they have to poop, telling you that they have to go prior to going in their diaper or starting to go in their pull up on a predictable daily schedule.

If your child is ready to potty train but isn't able to push out the stool, try having your child sit on the toilet backwards when trying. You can even give your child a dry erase marker and let them draw on the lid of the toilet seat while they have "Try Time." This is a good position for them to be in because it makes it easier for them to pass a bowel movement. Drawing on the toilet seat is silly and relaxing so will distract your child if they are stressed about trying to use the toilet.

Another fun thing to try that will help your child to learn to push to release a bowel movement, is to get bubbles or a balloon, and let your child blow while sitting on the toilet. This will help them to learn to bear down and push out the stool. Making toilet time as relaxed and happy as possible will help your child to be able to re-lax and go.

Even if your child isn't able to go during "Try Time" tell them that you are proud of them for trying. Normalize bowel movements as much as possible. Making too big of a deal out of them going, or not going, will add pressure and stress for both of you which will just delay the process.

If your child is using an adult toilet, I highly rec-ommend using a stool to raise their knees over the height of their hips. Squatty Potty is one common brand that works wonderfully. We are built to poop in a squatting position with our knees raised higher than out hips. This is espe-cially critical if your child's legs are dangling and their hips are tipped forward to be able to bal-ance on the toilet seat.

If your toddler is afraid of flushing, waiting until they are outside of the bathroom to flush can help. Gradually flush when they are closer to the toilet but don't rush them if they are stressed by it.

If your child has accidents, try to act as business-like and matter-of-act as possible about them. If you are upset, your child will feel the stress and it will make them nervous about going. Accidents are normal and should be treated as such. Constipation puts your child as risk of withholding their stool and any additional stress can make withholding even more likely.

Keeping anything potty related relaxed and fun will help your child to avoid or overcome withholding. Trying to potty train when a child is constipated can lead to them withholding. We'll go deeper into withholding in a future chapter.

Doing a clean-out for your constipated toddler can give you a clean slate to work on their constipation and get them having daily, smooth sausage like stools. Increasing magnesium until they pass a significant amount of stool will give you a clean slate, helps shrink down their bowels and will help you to keep a consistent dose so they have enough stool come out daily.

Any time you suspect that your toddler is becoming backed up, it is a good idea to give more magnesium, increase the amount of liquids they are drinking and oil they are eating to keep things moving. We'll go into more detail on all of these options in future chapters.

How to do a Constipation Clean Out for your child

If your child is severely constipated, has not passed any stool in 3 days, is bloated from stool backed up into their intestines, is trying to pass a bowel movement but nothing is coming out or only a few hard balls are coming out, is throwing up from being backed up or is very uncomfortable, it is time to do a clean out for your constipated child. A clean out can also be helpful when you are trying new treatments for your child's constipation so you can see what is working for them. After you have your child cleaned out, aim for 1-3 well formed stools a day.

I highly recommend tracking the dosing you are giving your child and their bowel movements when you do a clean-out. I have a free bowel movement tracker you can download. Go to this link for your free bowel movement tracker:

https://naturalconstipationsolutions.com/bowel-movement-tracker/

Many doctors recommend using Miralax (PEG 3350) or GoLYTELY (PEG 3350 with added electrolytes) for children as young as a few weeks old. Neither has been approved for use in children under 17. Over 30,000 reports of adverse events have been reported to the FDA from PEG 3350 use. Many families have reported that their children experienced tics, hallucinations, anxiety, OCD, panic attacks and seizures after a PEG 3350 clean out.

There are safe alternatives that you can use to help your child. If your child is hospitalized for a clean out, please research PEG 3350 and ask your child's doctor for other alternatives that are approved for pediatric use. Hospitals used magnesium citrate before Miralax was invented so that is a good alternative to ask about. Some magnesium citrate products still have PEG in them so always read the ingredients list prior to using.

Magnesium Citrate is generally recognized as safe and effective for use in children over 4. Natural Calm Magnesium Citrate is often used for children. I used it personally with my son when I was initially getting him off of Miralax years ago. His favorite was the lemon flavored.

You mix the Calm with hot water and it will fizz up which shows that it is activated, and then once it is done fizzing, add ice cold water. You can mix it into juice or lemonade instead of water if your child doesn't like it as is. They also make Natural Calm Gummies for children who don't like to drink flavored drinks.

If you want to use Natural Calm Magnesium Citrate for a clean-out for a child, what worked for my son was 1/2-1 tsp initial dose and then dosing an additional 1/2 tsp every two hours until you get loose stools. 1 Gummie is a similar amount of magnesium as 1/2 tsp of the regular Natural Calm.

The Natural Calm Powder comes in Original Flavor, Lemon, Raspberry Lemon, and Cherry. Calm is flavored with Stevia so it does have a different taste that might take some getting used to for some children. Or you might need to camouflage the flavor by mixing it with another drink. You can also use just a small amount of water to mix it and then use a syringe to get it in your child. Another option is to dilute the Calm with a lot of water until it is very mildly flavored. Then add a squeeze of lemon or lime or flavor with fruit or juice.

You can also get magnesium citrate as a pre-mixed drink that is almost like soda. It is important to always read the labels on these drinks because many of them contain polyethylene glycol, the only ingredient in Miralax. Sometimes one flavor by a company won't have PEG but another will, so you must check all of the labels to be sure what you are buying does not.

Every magnesium citrate drink I have looked at in drug stores have saccharine, which I avoid because it is a potential carcinogen. For a short-term clean out, it is still better than other options like Miralax, in my opinion.

Vitamin C can also be used for a clean out with children. Buffered vitamin C is more gentle on a child's stomach than other forms of Vitamin C and the powder can be mixed in their juice. Buffered Vitamin C also includes magnesium, calcium, and potassium so it is more balanced and less likely to cause problems than straight Vitamin C. Some kids do really well on a vitamin C flush. Vitamin C can cause gas and cramping plus the stool can be acidic and burn the skin on the child's bottom, so I recommend using coconut oil on their bottoms to prevent diaper rash or a sore bottom.

With children ages 1-3 years, start slowly with 30 mg of vitamin C and work up to 400 mg a day. For ages 4-8 years, you start at 40 mg and can go up to 650mg and for ages 9 and up, 1200 mg is the upper limit deemed safe by the Food and Nutrition Board of the Institute of Medicine. I would break up the vitamin C into small doses and dose every hour or two until you get loose stools.

When your child reaches bowel tolerance for magnesium or vitamin C there will be flushing from their bottom like after an enema. It may be hard for them to control and make it to the bathroom.

If your child is seriously impacted you may need to do a top-down (oral) and bottom-up (enemas or suppositories) program. Saline Enemas are safe for children 2-11. It isn't fun for you or for your child to do an enema but it may be what needs to happen to break up a hard ball of stool. If you are stressed about doing an enema, your child will sense this and it will make them stressed as well. Act as matter of fact as you can.

Have your child lay on his or her side on top of a towel on a soft surface. You can rub some coconut oil around the outside of your child's anus and then gently insert the tube into the anus. Aim towards the child's belly button. Gently squeeze the enema to flush the liquid into your child's colon. Have them lay there and hold the enema in for at least 5-10 minutes to give it time to work on softening up the hardball of stool. Then have them go to the potty and sit on the toilet to release the enema liquid and stool. It may take more than one to get the stool soft and moving.

Glycerine Suppositories will help lubricate the stool to come out easier. These are generally effective in producing a bowel movement in 15 minutes to one hour. The glycerine will soften and lubricate the stool to help your child expel it.

If your child has motility issues and you aren't having success with the other clean out methods, adding senna, either through a senna tea or with chocolate Ex-lax, can help them to go by causing the muscles in the intestines to contract. Senna is something you want to go easy with until you know how it will affect them. I also wouldn't recommend senna for long-term use as it can cause dependence but it is safer than many laxatives out there. The regular Ex-Lax pills have PEG so I would avoid them as well.

It is impossible for anyone to give you specific dosing information for your child. The Clean Out dosing isn't really based on age or size. It depends on how constipated your child is, how deficient your child is. Is there a hard ball of stool that needs to be broken up or does the child just have a lot of stool in the intestines? It will take experimentation and persistence to figure out what you need to do for your child to get them fully cleaned out.

I highly recommend trying anything you do for your child on yourself so you can see what they are experiencing, especially if they are non-verbal or low verbal.

Infants and Toddlers are harder to clean out safely. If your baby is in pain and seriously constipated I highly recommend taking your baby to a Functional or Integrative doctor or to a Naturopath and have them help you with a clean out and then help you to figure out why your infant is constipated.

Stopping solid foods for 24 hours might be enough to give your infant or toddler's gut time to move stool through. Just make sure to keep them hydrated during the 24 hour period with lots of water.

One safe solution that will help you to get your baby pooping is using a trace mineral supplement like <u>Omniblue Ocean Minerals</u>. It is safe for pregnant and nursing women and infants.

Dosing for infants and toddlers from the <u>Omniblue website</u>:

Infants and Toddlers Ages 1–4

The full-spectrum, pure-balanced OmniBlue magnesium and related trace elements are totally safe for infants to take for inducing regular bowel movements, unlike magnesium citrate which is not recommended for children under 4.

Start with 2–3 drops each feeding of soft infant foods, purees, soups and drinks regularly throughout the day until the point a bowel movement is induced, take note of the dosage and maintain the dosage.

Using an infant sized glycerine suppository will also help to lubricate and soften the stool making it easier to push out. If the suppository is too large, you can break off the back end of it to make it shorter for easier insertion. After you insert it, try to keep your baby or toddler's legs together for a few minutes to keep them from pushing it out before it dissolves.

Make sure your child, and if you are breastfeeding that you stay hydrated. You don't want your child to get dehydrated from the clean out. They will be expelling a lot of fluids during the clean out so you need them to drink even more than usual to keep them hydrated. A one-year-old should consume 8 ounces of water a day and the number of ounces should increase by 8 ounces for each year of age until reaching 8 years old or older when the child should be drinking at least 8, 8-ounce glasses of water a day.

Once your child is cleaned out, give them enough magnesium to ensure 1-3 bowel movements a day to prevent them from getting constipated again. Make sure that your child's stool is not hard, does not hurt when they pass it and ideally is a smooth sausage when they pass it. If they miss a day of going, up their magnesium. If their stool becomes harder, increase their magnesium. If they start passing liquid stools or can't hold their stool in until they reach the toilet, back off on the amount of magnesium you are giving them.

Magnesium for Constipation Relief

One of the quickest, safest and most effective ways to treat constipation without using a chemical laxative is with Magnesium. Most of us, and our kids, are magnesium deficient. Even if you are eating a healthy diet with lots of greens and other magnesium-rich foods, our soil is depleted of magnesium so our food is magnesium deficient. It is hard to get enough just by diet alone, especially if you don't have an ideal diet.

I have had people tell me that they have tried magnesium for their constipation and it didn't work for them. When I ask them how much and how often they took magnesium, they often say that they took one dose, one time. If you are magnesium deficient, your body is going to hold on to the magnesium to try to keep as much as possible. It may take many doses, and more than the normal dose, to produce a bowel movement or do a clean out. Parents are often surprised at how much magnesium it is taking to get their child to go.

You may think that your child had a blood test and it didn't come back magnesium deficient so this can't be their issue but only 1% of magnesium is stored in the blood. The rest is in your bones and organs. Blood tests for magnesium deficiency aren't very reliable or accurate.

Signs of magnesium deficiency are fatigue, muscle weakness, cramps or spasms, or even heart palpitations. Magnesium deficiency can trigger panic attacks, anxiety, diabetes, depression, migraine, liver or kidney problems, PCOS, fibromyalgia, asthma and of course, constipation. So you can see that getting enough is really important.

Magnesium works as an osmotic. It pulls water into the colon softening the stool. When you get too much magnesium, the stool is very soft or liquid and you expel the stool and the extra magnesium. No matter what type of magnesium you use, it can cause dehydration, so please make sure to drink lots of fluids.

There are many types of magnesium. Magnesium in supplements are generally bound to another ion. What the magnesium is bound to, impacts how much your child's body will absorb.

The type of magnesium you should use depends on your goal. With a constipated child, we have two goals. Our first goal is to use magnesium to produce regular bowel movements. Our second goal is to increase the magnesium stores in our child's body, so our child is no longer magnesium deficient.

Milk of Magnesia is magnesium hydroxide. It works as an antacid in addition to being a form of magnesium. Using anything that acts as an antacid isn't something I really think is a good idea for regular use. Many of our children are dealing with having low stomach acid, reflux, GERD etc, so reducing stomach acid, even more, is going to cause worsening symptoms. We need acid to digest our food and kill off harmful bacteria and pathogens.

If you are using Milk of Magnesia, make sure it only has magnesium hydroxide and water as the ingredients. Many have mineral oil which is a petroleum product, saccharin or even a bleaching agent like sodium hypochlorite. None of which are ingredients you want in your child. If you are having success with it, make sure to work on other ways to increase stomach acids like Apple Cider Vinegar or lemon water and make sure your child drinks a lot of water.

Magnesium sulfate or Epsom salt can be used internally, by mouth for the laxative effect or used in a bath, where it is absorbed through the skin. This is a great option because we need sulfur too and magnesium sulfate is a great way to get magnesium and sulfur. It can be harder to get kids to take it by mouth due to its taste but some parents have had success mixing a small amount in juice or with honey for children over 12 months.

Epsom salt baths are one of my favorite things to do for a constipated child. The skin absorbs the magnesium sulfate and the child is often relaxed by the warm water and the magnesium and will often have to jump out of the tub to have a bowel movement or *warning!* have a bowel movement in the tub. You want an Epsom salt that is listed with directions for laxative use. If it has directions for laxative use you know it is safe to take by mouth or use in the tub. Not all epsom salts are safe to be taken by mouth, either because they are not pure epsom salt or because they have additives like scents.

Magnesium citrate has a long history of being used for constipation and is usually well tolerated by children. Magnesium citrate is what was used for colonoscopy preparation or Clean Outs before Polyethylene Glycol (Miralax, PEG 3350 or Golightly) was invented. Magnesium citrate isn't well absorbed so it isn't the best way to correct a deficiency but it is a great way to induce a bowel movement. It usually works in 1-3 hours, but can take overnight or if your child is severely constipated. It might also take multiple doses over days to break up hard stool in your child's intestines. Magnesium citrate can be used for Clean Outs and to get your child going daily to shrink the bowels while you are looking for the root cause of their constipation.

Many of the bottles of liquid magnesium citrate have PEG (polyethylene glycol) or saccharine in them. They are flavored and are kind of like soda so some kids will drink them easier than other options. I try to avoid Saccharine because it is a neurotoxin and a carcinogen. I would avoid those if at all possible but they are still a better option than many over the counter laxatives. Using them occasionally for a clean out is probably not going to cause long term issues but I wouldn't use them regularly.

Natural Calm Magnesium is a good brand of Magnesium citrate that also comes in child friendly flavors like lemon or raspberry lemon. They taste like lemonade or pink lemonade. You need to add a small amount of very hot water to the Calm powder to activate it and then once the fizzing stops, add water, ice, juice, lemonade etc. It has stevia for a sweetener, the taste of which can take some getting used to. You can add honey or sugar as well if your child doesn't like the taste. You can dilute the Calm in a large drink as long as your child will drink that much or you can just add a small amount of water and put it in your child's mouth with a syringe if they really don't like the taste.

I have used Natural Calm and have had good success getting my super-taster son to take it. I add in cut up lemons or limes and put in lots of ice after activating it with hot to boiling water. Some of my readers have had good luck freezing it after they mix it up in Popsicle molds. Natural Calm is now selling a Gummie which kids really seem to like and the gummies can be a great way to get magnesium in your child if they won't drink anything flavored or take pills. You can also make a slushy with Calm after you mix it up adding ice, lemonade or limeade and blend it up. Some kids will drink it that way that won't drink it straight up.

Magnesium oxide isn't absorbed well so it doesn't work for magnesium deficiency but does work to produce bowel movements short term. Magnesium oxide also works as an antacid like Magnesium hydroxide. We need acid to digest our food, so while it works short term as a laxative, long-term it can prevent you from properly digesting your food. Low stomach acid can contribute to constipation so I wouldn't recommend it for long-term use. I generally don't recommend using Magnesium oxide for more than a couple of days to produce a bowel movement.

Omniblue Ocean Minerals contain magnesium along with other minerals that your body needs including potassium, sulfate, and sodium. It has a strong salty taste that can be tricky to camouflage but it is a really well-rounded supplement that won't cause an electrolyte imbalance. This is a great option for adults and if your child is willing to take it, it is a great option for them as well. It is especially good for maintenance and to correct mineral deficiencies.

Dosing suggestions from the Omniblue website.[1]

For Nursing Mothers and Babies

Add one or two drops to infant's formula or pumped milk for each feeding. The minerals will absorb perfectly into the formula and milk and at these levels will induce a natural rhythmic release of the bowels. Monitor the number of drops per feeding for your baby for the point where they regulate the bowels and then maintain that level.

Infants and Toddlers Ages 1–4

The full-spectrum, pure-balanced OmniBlue magnesium and related trace elements are totally safe for infants to take for inducing regular bowel movements, unlike magnesium citrate which is not recommended for children under 4.

Start with 2–3 drops each feeding of soft infant foods, purees, SOUPS and drinks regularly throughout the day until the point a bowel movement is induced, take note of the dosage and maintain the dosage. Not only are you cre-

---

[1] https://omniblueminerals.com/

ating healthy bowel movements but full-spectrum minerals are necessary every day for everybody as the fundamental fuel and cell activation for the body to function at its highest levels.

Children Ages 5-8

¼ teaspoon distributed throughout their daily meals. The minerals at smaller regular doses will mix in with food flavors perfectly and you can also cook with these minerals! Add to salad dressings, soups, and any sauces, very low sodium.

Children 9-13

½ teaspoon distributed throughout their daily meals taking note where the dose stimulates their natural bowel movement. This may vary more or less from 1/2 teaspoon depending on body weight and metabolism. This is totally safe and these doses should be maintained anyway not only to regulate the bowels naturally but also because they are essential daily for everyone's health.

Younger Adults 14–18

Between ½ and 1 teaspoon daily distributed with foods and drinks.

Magnesium malate is very absorbable. This is a great form if you are trying to correct a magnesium deficiency. Your body will hold on to more of the magnesium. But this type doesn't necessarily work as well to get a bowel movement because it does absorb really well into your bodies cells. Your body won't flush out the extra with a bowel movement because it is able to use the magnesium you are giving it. But it will build up your child's magnesium stores so if you use other magnesium supplements in conjunction, like citrate, you will need less Magnesium citrate to get a bowel movement after a while as you build up the magnesium in your system.

Magnesium chloride can be taken orally, or used in the tub or as a magnesium oil which is applied topically. You can use magnesium oil by rubbing it on the skin or rubbing it into the soles of the feet. It can sting when you apply it to the skin so mixing it with coconut oil or another carrier oil can help it to not sting as much. Magnesium Chloride taken internally can help boost stomach acid so it a good option if your child has reflux, GERD or low stomach acid. It is hard to hide it in foods or drinks as it has a strong taste but is well absorbed through the skin. Because it is well absorbed it is less likely to work well for constipation relief or a clean out.

Magnesium L-Threonate is a newer magnesium supplement. It is showing promise for absorption and for penetrating the cell membranes. This would be a good choice to build up your magnesium stores but doesn't work as well if you are using it for constipation.

Magnesium glycinate is excellent for magnesium deficiencies but not the best for constipation.

I would avoid Magnesium stearate as a supplement.

With any magnesium supplement, it may take a higher dose thank you would expect to get to the point of loose stools. When someone is deficient, the body will grab on to the magnesium and hold onto it. So you need to keep dosing until you get loose stools. It is tempting to do a dose or two and throw in the towel and say it didn't work. But it will work, you just need to find what the bowel's tolerance is for magnesium and the more deficient you are, the higher that tolerance will be.

A question I get daily is "How much Magnesium do I need to give my child. He is X years old and Y pounds." Every child is different. Some small children are very deficient and need more than an adult. How much magnesium you will need to use to produce a bowel movement often depends more on how deficient your child is in magnesium than how old they are or how much they weigh. Different types of magnesium work differently in different children.

The way to figure out your child's dosage is to dose them with a small amount every two hours until you get loose stools. The next day give less than the total you gave the day before that caused them to have loose stools. The dosing can change over time as they build up magnesium in their system. If they get loose stools, lower the dose slightly. If their stool is hard or they miss a day, increase the dose the next day.

Don't wait to dose until your child hasn't gone for a few days. Dose daily to keep things moving so you don't end up dealing with an impaction.

I personally like to use a mix of many types of magnesiums, to build up your child's store of magnesium and to relieve constipation.

Finding the amount of magnesium that works for your child can be a moving target because the amount needed to reach bowel tolerance can change over time as you rebuild your magnesium stores.

Taking an Epsom salt bath, rubbing magnesium cream on your tummy or feet and taking Natural Calm might all be needed in the beginning to keep your child regular. In addition to magnesium, you need to make sure you don't get your calcium, D3 and K2 out of whack so if you are supplementing with magnesium it is good to supplement with these as well.

Talk to your child's doctor about their recommendations for magnesium supplementation. Unfortunately, some doctors don't have a lot of education in magnesium supplementation so they aren't comfortable with it. A Functional or Integrative doctor will be more likely to have the knowledge to help you with magnesium supplementation.

In addition to supplements, adding magnesium-rich foods is a great way to build up your magnesium store. Leafy greens, seaweed, pumpkin seeds, almonds, Brazil nuts or cashews, and cocoa powder are all good options to get magnesium from food.

Magnesium is needed for so many things in our body that even if your child isn't constipated any longer, it is good to continue to be aware of how much magnesium they are getting through their diet and supplements.

Other Over-the-Counter Remedies for Constipation Relief

There are many safe and effective over the counter supplements that you can use to help your child have a bowel movement quickly and easily.

Senna

Senna is an herbal laxative made from the leaves and fruit of the senna plant. If your child has motility issues and struggles to push out their stool then senna can be helpful in the initial stages of getting your child to have 1-3 bowel movements a day. The main ingredient in Ex-lax chocolates isSenna. Senna causes cramping. It works by irritating the lining of the bowel. This can be uncomfortable for most children but for children with motility issues it can help them to push out their stool. Usually, you take Senna before bed, it works overnight and produces a bowel movement the next morning.

Avoid Ex-lax pills as they have polyethylene glycol, the only ingredient in Miralax. Over 25,000 reports of adverse events have been made to the FDA for Polyethylene Glycol including pediatric deaths. I do not ever recommend using Miralax or any products that contain PEG/Polyethylene Glycol. Smooth is also Senna and is also an excellent option for a stimulant laxative in children. Senna is not for long-term use because it causes dependency and if you use it with your child for too long, your child will not be able to go without it.

Vitamin C
When you get too much Vitamin C, your body expels the excess similar to how it does with magnesium. You can mix buffered Vitamin C with water if your child will take it that way or mix it with a little bit of water and then mix that in with your child's favorite juice. You could make a slushee with this as well. Using a fun straw, or a fancy cup is always a good way to encourage your child to drink.

If your child is older, and can swallow pills, Vitamin C tablets are a good option. C-Salts are a form of Vitamin C that is buffered so stomach friendly. It also has some magnesium and potassium which are helpful for constipation. This is a powder so you can mix it in water or juice. It is effervescent, so if your child likes soda or other fizzy drinks, this might be a good choice. Some kids don't like anything with fizz so this wouldn't work for them. It is non-GMO with no fillers.

In some kids, taking Vitamin C for constipation works really well, but for some, it causes very acidic stool which leads to burning when the child has a bowel movement and rashes from the acidic stool touching your child's skin.

With children ages 1-3, start slowly with 30 mg and work up to 400mg a day. For ages 4-8 years you start at 40 mg and can go up to 650mg and for 9 and up, 1200mg is the upper limit deemed safe by the Food and Nutrition Board of the Institute of Medicine. I would break up the Vitamin C into small doses and dose every hour until you get loose stools. After you figure out what dose causes loose stools, give your child slightly less than that in the future to keep them going daily.

Salt
We have been taught to be scared of salt, but the first thing that happens when you go to the hospital is they put you on a saline (salt water) drip. We need salt. Salt is necessary for many of the chemical reactions that support enzyme function, hormone production, and protein transport. But we need high-quality salt with trace minerals. Not table salt that has aluminum and is bleached. New research is showing that low sodium diets are not good for people. Even people with high blood pressure need high quality salt in their diet.

You can use a high-quality salt like Celtic Sea Salt (my personal choice) or Himalayan for constipation relief. Do not use table salt which may be bleached and have aluminum in it.

Celtic Sea Salt has over 80 trace minerals in addition to the sodium. It is non-GMO, Kosher, Gluten Free and doesn't have any caking agents. We used Himalayan salt for a while but found the Celtic Sea Salt to work much better for our health and it tastes amazing. Mixing salt into a glass of water and drinking until you get loose stools is one way, but a tastier way to ingest salt is with my electrolyte drink.

Electrolyte Drink

I cup orange juice
1/2 to 1 tsp of Celtic sea salt
1/4 Tsp organic Epsom salt (magnesium)
1/8 tsp non GMO cream159 of tartar (potassium)
1 cup to 1 1/2 cups of cold water, depending on taste

Make sure the brand of Epsom salt you buy has directions for laxative use so you know it is safe to take by mouth.

It is very refreshing and it also has a very strong laxative effect. It usually starts to work in minutes but you can drink multiple recipes worth if it doesn't work right away or you are attempting to do a clean out. It may take 4 ounces or 4 recipes worth depending on how deficient in salt and minerals your child is.

You might need to start with a lower amount of the ingredients and work up to the level that works for your child or try different ratios for your child. This is a very flexible recipe.

Oils

Ingesting oil is a great way to lubricate the stool and help poop to pass easily, especially if you have old, hard stool in the intestines.

I believe that castor oil is safer for short term use for constipation relief than mineral oil but neither one should be used for more than 7 days.

Castor oil has been used medically for thousands of years. There is evidence of it being used by ancient Egyptians. Generations of mothers have used Castor oil for constipation relief for their families. When something has been used for thousands of years, it generally shows that it is safe and effective. Castor oil is considered "generally regarded as safe" by the FDA. Castor oil works as a stimulant laxative when taken internally. Castor oil is 90% ricinoleic acid. The ricinoleic acid causes smooth muscle contractions in your intestines pushing the stool through your intestines and helping you to have a bowel movement.

Mineral oil works by lubricating the stool to help it pass through your intestines and it also coats it to increase the fluid in the stool making it easier to pass. It is a petroleum product. It is a by-product of the distillation of petroleum to become gasoline. There is concern that mineral oil contains contaminants that could affect our health and may even contribute to cancer. Personally, I avoid any products that are petroleum based.

There is also a risk of aspiration when taking mineral oil by mouth. This is especially concerning in young children and anyone who is bedridden. If you do decide to use mineral oil, look for one with directions for laxative use on the package. Mineral oil can also cause anal leakage or uncontrollable diarrhea.

Castor oil is very effective for constipation relief and is generally safe for most people. Taking Castor oil internally repeatedly can cause potassium deficiency. If your child has heart issues then I would not use it or if your child develops a rash, discontinue use.

Side effects from using castor oil internally can include cramping and digestive upset. Do not use if pregnant or breastfeeding. Consult your physician for recommendations on castor oil use for your particular situation.

When you take castor oil internally it works fairly quickly, usually within 2-6 hours so do not give too closely to bedtime as it will interrupt your child's sleep with them needing to use the bathroom multiple times. It causes very strong contractions and the urge to go. It can be difficult to make it to the restroom when you take it internally.

Coconut oil is my favorite oil for constipation in children. It is more palatable for children than many other oil options and can be added to their diet in many child-friendly ways.

Coconut oil is rich in Medium Chain Fatty Acids. MCFA's boost your metabolism which makes the stool pass through your intestines faster, the oil coats and lubricates harder old stool making it easier to pass and it softens the newly formed stool making it easier to pass.

There are many ways to use coconut oil. Instead of using other oils in your cooking or baking, you can use coconut oil. You can use it instead of butter on toast or veggies. Some kids just eat it directly off the spoon. It has a mild, almost sweet flavor.

But, it can be tricky to get enough coconut oil into children who are struggling with constipation. It can be especially difficult for children with sensory issues or autism or ones who just don't like the taste of coconut oil. One of the easiest ways I have found to get children to eat enough coconut oil to relieve constipation is with Chocolate Coconut Oil Poop Candy.

To make **Poop Candy**, you want to use equal parts chocolate chips to coconut oil. 1 cup to 1 cup or 1/2 cup to 1/2 cup. If you are going to make a lot of these, a double boiler is really handy. If you don't have one, you can make a makeshift double boiler with a Pyrex bowl over a pan. Add a couple of inches of water to the pan, put the bowl over the pan and then heat on low heat while stirring the chocolate/coconut oil mixture until it melts. Once it is smooth and lump free, pour it into a silicone candy mold. I add a sprinkle of course ground Celtic Sea Salt to the mold before I pour in the chocolate.

Carefully put the filled mold in the refrigerator or freezer until the chocolates are firm. The silicone molds can bend so it often helps to put the mold on a plate before you add the chocolate so you can carry it to the fridge without spilling it. It usually takes less than 30 minutes for them to harden depending on the size of the mold. Then pop the chocolates out and serve.

The chocolates that are left over need to be stored in the fridge or freezer. They melt quickly and can be messy. My son isn't much of a sweet eater but he loves these.

If your child doesn't like chocolate you can use any nut or seed butter instead of the chocolate chips or you can use candy melts or add in ground flax meal, shredded coconut, or dried nuts or seeds to change the texture.

I would start out slowly with just one or two depending on the size of your mold (The mold I use is about an inch across and my son eats two at a time) and then have a couple every two hours until your child goes. Coconut oil can cause very loose stools if you eat a lot of it. That can be a benefit, or not so much, depending on what your goal is.

Stress-free Suppositories and Enemas for Your Child

Using a suppository or enema isn't fun for you or for your child but it may be what needs to happen to break up a hard ball of stool. There are things that you can do to make it stress-free for yourself and for your child.

Enemas and suppositories are especially useful when your child hasn't gone in a few days and has hard stool lower down in their intestines. The suppository or enema will soften and lubricate the stool, making it easier to pass. Enemas go further up into the colon so they are more effective for more severe backups.

If you are stressed about doing an enema or inserting a suppository, your child will sense this and it will make them stressed as well. Act as matter of fact as you can.

If it makes you feel better, you can wear latex or nitrile gloves. If your child is older, ask them if they have any suggestions on how they would like the process to go. Including them in the process will make it easier for both of you.

If you have never done a suppository or enema on yourself, I highly recommend giving yourself one before giving your child one so you know what they are experiencing. They will also respect that you are on the same team and you can give them a detailed explanation of how it worked and what it felt like. If you are comfortable with it, you can even have your child in the room with you when you do your enema so they can see that there isn't anything to fear and that you aren't hurt.

Warm everything to just above body temperature so it doesn't jolt them when you put it in, give your child electronics to distract them or turn on the TV and if you think it will help them, explain to them the steps you will be doing so they aren't worried about what is coming next. Explain to your child how much better they will feel once the old poop comes out. If they are fearful, it can help them to show them the steps of the procedure on a doll.

Older children might be interested in giving the suppository or enema to themselves. Having this control might make them feel better about the process. If so, then talk them through what needs to happen and stand by to give direction.

If your child is a teen and embarrassed to have you help them with the enema, sit down and discuss the process, ask them to explain it back to you so you know they understand what needs to happen so they can do it on their own. If they don't want you in the room, you can offer to have them put you on speaker phone on their phone so they can ask you questions but still maintain privacy.

Suppositories

Pediatric sized glycerine suppositories are safe for children ages 2-6 and will help lubricate the stool to come out easier. Adult sized glycerine suppositories are usually ok for children 6 and up. (read directions on the box to be sure) The glycerine will soften and lubricate the stool to help your child expel it. These are generally effective in producing a bowel movement in 15 minutes to one hour. The longer your child can keep it in, the more effective it will be.

If you are having a hard time getting the suppository in your child's anus, you can shave the suppository down smaller so it is easier to insert, just make sure that it isn't too pointy. You don't want it to poke your child and hurt them.

Suppositories aren't going to go as deep as an enema, so might be easier for some parents to give to their kids but they also won't break up a large hard stool as well as an enema.

Suppositories can cause a burning sensation in your child's rectum so if your child is uncomfortable, this isn't unusual but can make your child worried or scared. Coating it in coconut oil or another lubricant can help.

Enemas

Enemas work better, on severely constipated children, than suppositories. If your child hasn't had a bowel movement in many days or is very dehydrated causing the stool to become dry and hard or is not able to pass their stool because the stool is too large and hard to push out, then an enema might be a better option for you. The enema solution will travel 12-24 inches up into your child loosening up their stool so it is much more effective if your child is severely constipated.

To do an enema on your child, have your child lay on his or her side on top of a towel or a chuck pad on a soft surface with their knees bent up at a 90-degree angle. You can rub some coconut oil or another lubricant around the outside of your child's anus and the tip of the enema to make it easier to insert the enema.

Make sure all of the air has been pushed out of the enema bulb or bag before inserting.

Warm the tip up with your hands beforehand. Cold can make muscles tense and make using the enema on your child more stressful for them.

Gently insert the enema tube into the anus 1 1/2 to 2 inches. Aim towards the child's belly button. If you feel any resistance, stop and back off. You do not want to push and puncture their colon. Slowly and gently wiggle the tip a bit and insert again. You don't need to get in very deep for it to be effective.

Gently and slowly squeeze the enema bulb to flush the liquid into your child's colon. If you are using an enema bag, raise the bag above your child and let gravity push the fluid in.

Once you have the enema solution in your child's colon, remove the enema device and have your child lay there and hold the enema in for 2-20 minutes to give it time to work on softening up the hard ball of stool. If your child is having a hard time holding it in, you can help by putting gentle pressure on the outside of their bottom to squeeze their cheeks together or have your child blow out like they are blowing bubbles.

The longer they can keep the enema liquid in, the more effective it will be. If they are feeling a strong urge to have a bowel movement or at the end of the amount of time you have chosen, let them go and sit on the potty to release the enema and stool.

It may take more than one enema to get the stool soft and moving if they are severely

75

backed up and haven't gone for many days. The harder the stool is, the longer it will take for the enema solution to soften it.

There are multiple types of enemas. Glycerine, saline, soap suds, and milk and molasses enemas are the most common ones used in children.

You can buy packaged pediatric sized saline and glycerine enemas at the drug store. They are one-time use and disposable, making them easy to do and you have no clean up.

Milk and molasses enema are very effective and are used by hospitals and ER's for clean-outs on constipated children with great success. To do a Milk and Molasses enema use equal parts of milk and molasses. Warm the milk to 105-110 degrees and mix the molasses in until it is all blended together. Use a rectal enema bulb or enema kit which you can get at the pharmacy or order online.

Soap Suds enemas are made with distilled water and a liquid Castile soap, like Dr. Bronner's. Use 1 tsp to 1 Tbs of Castile soap per cup of distilled water. This enema works by irritating the lining of the colon, the more soap you use, the more irritation it will cause. I would start out with a smaller amount of soap and increase if it doesn't work for your child. Heat the distilled water and soap mixture to 105-110 degrees and then use the solution in an enema bulb syringe or enema bag kit.

If you do not have success with one enema solution or your child doesn't like it, try a different one until you find one that is effective and comfortable for your child.

Enemas and suppositories can cause dependence if used regularly. But some doctors do recommend daily use of enemas for children who withhold, wet the bed due to chronic constipation, have motility issues, encopresis, congenital Megacolon or a stretched out colon from being chronically constipated, to allow the colon to shrink back down in size and regain sensation. Discuss enemas and suppositories with your child's doctor if you feel that they might help your child if used daily long-term if your child has any of these issues where enema or suppository use might be necessary.

If you are using a reusable enema bulb or enema bag, everything must be thoroughly cleaned. After use, disassemble the parts as much as possible. Wash in a solution of Castile soap and water or vinegar and water. The bag just needs to be rinsed with water. You can also flush the enema tip, tube or bulb with hydrogen peroxide if you are concerned about leaving any germs behind. Make sure to wash all of the cleaning solutions out with tap water and let air dry.

Enemas can be dehydrating so make sure your child drinks a lot of liquids after you complete the enema process. If you are regularly using enemas, the enemas can wash out the beneficial bacteria from your child's colon. I highly recommend adding in a high quality probiotic to your child's regimen.

Enemas and suppositories are effective but they are a short term solution to chronic constipation. For a long term solution, you need to work on figuring out why your child is constipated.

Withholding - When Your Child is Afraid to Poop

There isn't much that is more frustrating than to see that your child has to go to the bathroom and that they are doing everything in their power to hold it in. Most kids withhold occasionally. Often, they withhold because they are busy playing and don't want to stop and take time out to go to the bathroom. We remind them to go and they fuss a bit and then go.

But when withholding is a chronic issue it can be a huge problem that takes over your life and gets progressively worse over time. When your child holds their stool until the urge to go is gone repeatedly, the stool will eventually get very large, dried out and even harder to push out. This causes a horrible cycle of the child fearing to go because of the pain, and by holding, they make it more painful to go in the future, confirming to them that pooping hurts so they hold it more.

There are ways to break this cycle.

Why do children chronically withhold their stool? In most cases, it is because it hurts to go. We

79

have a biological urge to move our bowels. When you feel that urge and have to hold it for some reason, it is really uncomfortable. There is a reason why a child would do that instead of just pooping and feeling better. They aren't doing it to be difficult or because they are stubborn or trying to upset you.

Often it hurts to go because the child is or was constipated and there was pain when he went so he's afraid to go again and have it hurt.

Part of the solution is to get poops soft so they don't hurt. That isn't always enough for some children because they have learned that poop hurts and is scary. It may take months to get past the fear even after their constipation resolves but it is possible.

Chronic Withholding usually starts out as a constipation issue and transitions into a behavioral issue.

First, you have to work on solving your child's constipation. You are looking to get their stool to a pudding or applesauce consistency so they have no pain pushing it out. If they are still resistant, you can up the magnesium, or whatever you are using, until the stool is so liquid that they can't hold it.

After you find something that is helping your child to have soft, pain-free poops, then it is time to address the behavioral issues involved in withholding.

Kids feed off of our anxiety. The more they hold their poop, the more anxious we get about them pooping. This gives the kids a tremendous amount of power over the family because they get a ton of attention for not pooping.

It is important to normalize pooping as much as possible. Take him or her in with you when you have to use the toilet. Have other family members take him in with them when they poop so he can see it is normal and doesn't hurt. Have a toy car or "dude" or doll poop. There are toys and dolls that eat and poop. These can be helpful toys for children who withhold. You can encourage them to "potty train" their toy or change their doll's diaper after they "go." If you have pets, you can discuss your pet going and praise them for having a bowel movement. Encourage your child to praise your pet for going to the bathroom. Modeling pooping can really help with young children, whether they watch people, animals or toys go.

Often, potty training brings on withholding. Your child might not be developmentally ready to go on a toilet, even if they are peeing on the toilet. We are in a hurry to get them out of diapers for deadlines set by preschools or daycare providers but if your child isn't developmentally ready to learn to poop on the potty, pushing for it can really set them backward and turn withholding into a chronic problem. If you can, back off of toilet training completely and revisit it down the road when you are past the withholding.

Hopefully, you can work with your daycare or preschool provider to take the pressure off of toilet training until your child is ready. It might take a doctor's note in some cases to accomplish this. Also, if your child is going on the toilet but is struggling with toileting issues, ask his or her teacher to not put limits on your child when he or she asks to use the restroom.

Having a teacher tell your child that they need to wait until a restroom break or shame them for not being able to hold it, can compound issues with withholding. You can also talk to your child's teachers about your child having access to a private one stall restroom such as the bathroom at the nurse's office if going in public is difficult for him or her. For older children who withhold, you can request a 504 plan be put in place in their school for toileting issues if you have a medical reason for it. I would work with your child's pediatrician to get the necessary information for your child's school to set up a 504 plan for them.

When you back off of toilet training for pooping you can still make incremental steps towards potty training that aren't as stressful but will help you to make progress. If your child is squatting in the living room in their pull up, encourage them to go into the bathroom to go. Or encourage them to sit on the potty in their diaper even if they don't go. It will make the toilet much less scary.

Make sitting on the toilet a positive experience. Read to your child, let them have electronics that they usually can't have or let them watch videos that they only get to watch on the potty. Limit the "try times" to just a few minutes. You don't want them to view sitting on the potty as a punishment so limit it to just 4 or 5 minutes. Tell them "thank you" for trying. You can make a sticker chart for "trying" but don't do such elaborate rewards that it builds up trying or going in their head too much. It should be more of an acknowledgment of accomplishment than a bribe. Although, with some kids, a bribe really works too!

Reading books about using the toilet can be very interesting for some children and also help to normalize the experience. Look for books about animals that feature information about digestion and pooping to help your child become comfortable with the concept.

For older children, The Magic School Bus has an episodes that talk about digestion. You can buy DVD's or find the individual episodes on youtube.

Sometimes, changing the language we use can make a huge difference in how our child perceives a stressful situation. Instead of asking your child go to the bathroom you can talk about getting his or her oil changed or joke about the bathroom being the spa where they get Epsom salt baths, and massages on their tummy. Make the bathroom a happy place instead of a place of stress. The more anxiety you have about your child going, the more he or she will have. I know that is hard! But if you have anxiety, he will sense it and it will make him think that there is something to fear.

If you know that it doesn't hurt your child to poop any longer, then you might want to get some edible glitter (not because you are going to eat it but so it doesn't mess up your plumbing!) You can have your child put a pinch of the glitter in the toilet and tell him or her that it is magic glitter and makes it easy and pain-free to poop. If your child is still struggling with some pain I wouldn't do this or your child will not have any faith that it will help.

If your child has moved from a potty training chair to a regular toilet and is struggling then there are some things you can do to help them to relax and be able to go.

We are actually built to squat to poop. Sitting on a toilet can make it harder to push out the poop. Especially if you are little and your bottom feels like it is going to fall into the water and your feet don't touch the floor and are just swinging. Getting a potty seat that fits on the toilet and a potty stool like a Squatty Potty can make a huge difference in your child being able to push out their stool. Ideally, your child's knees should be higher than the height of their hips. Some families have had success with their child standing on the toilet seat and squatting down with their support. That might not be a long-term fix but it might be something to try.

Core strength can make it hard for some kids to push out the stool. They might not be intentionally withholding in the beginning but not strong enough to push out a stool if they get mildly constipated. If your child has been diagnosed with Low Tone, then working on core strength, along with making their stool soft, can really help them with potty training and withholding.

One thing that we have had great success with is a mini-trampoline. It helps to build up your child's core so they can push better. Plus it is great for anxiety, sensory issues and just plain fun. We have had a mini trampoline in our living room for years and we joke that it bounces down the poop!

Having your child sit backwards on the toilet can also help them to have more leverage to push as they can lean forward and hold onto the back of the seat or the toilet tank. Many families have found that having their child blow bubbles or blow up a balloon while on the toilet can help the child to isolate the muscles they need to use to push out the poop. For older children, blowing up balloons can help them to isolate the muscles that push out the poop and help them to get the poop to come out.

Epsom salt or magnesium chloride baths are a wonderful way to relax your child and also the magnesium sulfate in the Epsom salt or the magnesium chloride absorb through their skin and can help them to go.

Doing silly crab walks where you both squat down and race across the living room in a crouched position can help your child to feel the urge to go and will get them in a position where the colon is positioned correctly for the stool to come out. Doing a dance party with them and as you turn the music down, everyone slowly crouches down and when the music gets turned louder everyone slowing comes back to standing can also help build strength and position the colon.

Some children who withhold when they are awake, end up going in their sleep. As frustrating as that is, it is good that they are going and getting the poop out. I recommend getting disposable underpads and putting them under your child when they sleep or letting them sleep in pull-ups or night time pull ups if they are older.

If they go in the night, try to be very matter of fact, tell them that you are just glad they went. Change the underpad and whatever else you need to and then move on.   If they feel ashamed or embarrassed it will just set the process back even more and cause everyone more stress. And it really is good that the poop came out before it got harder and then caused them pain, continuing the cycle of withholding. You can remind them that pooping doesn't hurt because if it did, it would have woken them up when they went.

Megacolon, motility issues, Hirschsprung's and nerve damage can all cause behaviors that look like withholding but are actually structural issues that prevent your child from feeling that they have to go or going easily or fully. If you aren't making progress, then I suggest going to a Functional or Integrative Medicine Doctor or Naturopath and having them help you to figure out if there is something medical that is keeping your child from going.

My son has Megacolon. Miralax didn't help him with going and caused lasting damage. As we got his constipation under control with natural methods and his gut healed, he gained back the sensation that tells him when he has to go.

If your child has blood in his or her stool, especially if it is black, then I would take your child to the doctor. If your child has red in his or her stool, then that can mean that he or she has hemorrhoid or a fissure. Try using coconut oil internally, on the anus and adding it to their diet to make the stools softer and easier to pass. Witch Hazel can help soothe and heal hemorrhoids, making it less painful to go.

Epsom salt baths are very soothing for these hemorrhoids as well. Fissures are actual tears in the colon and are aggravated by constipation. Keeping the stool very soft is critical in healing them. It may take months to get them to heal completely.

There is no quick solution to withholding but you will figure out what works for your child and eventually, this will not be an issue that you are dealing with any longer. Don't give up hope! You will get there. It takes a lot of patience and a good supportive team where everyone is working together for the benefit of your child.

If you have doctors pushing you to use Miralax or other laxatives, there are other safer and more effective, alternatives and there are also better doctors who will help you figure out why your child is withholding. A good doctor will help you to get to the root cause of your child's constipation and withholding issues instead of just putting a toxic band-aid over the problem and then sending you home to deal with it on your own.

Finding the Root Cause of Your Child's Constipation

Gluten is a Common Cause of Constipation

One of the most common causes of constipation in children is gluten. Gluten is a protein in grains including wheat, barley, rye, and triticale. Oats can also be an issue for people who have Celiac or gluten intolerance. Both Celiac and Non-Celiac Gluten Sensitivity can cause health issues, including constipation.

Many doctors are under the misconception that Celiac and Gluten Intolerance only cause diarrhea so if you report that your child is constipated, they don't always think of Celiac and don't test for Celiac. My own son struggled with constipation and was diagnosed with Celiac through a blood test at 18 months.

Some signs of gluten intolerance or Celiac are bloating, diarrhea, constipation, excessively bad smelling stools, pale colored stools, abdominal pain, headaches including migraines, fatigue, rashes (Dermatitis Herpetiformis, Eczema, Psoriasis, Alopecia and Chronic Urticaria) depression, weight loss or failure to thrive, iron deficiency anemia, anxiety and joint or muscle pain or brain fog.

A bloated tummy is very common in children with Celiac or Non-Celiac Gluten Sensitivity. You can see that her arms and legs are slim but her tummy is very distended and swollen. If your child's tummy is swollen like this, even if they have no other symptoms, I would get him or her tested for Celiac.

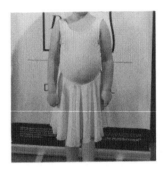 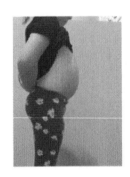

When my son was a baby, he had horribly smelly stools. They smelled so badly that if I was changing his diaper upstairs you could smell it all across the house and downstairs. The smell would hang in the air after. It smelled rancid like the stool had fermented in him. And to an extent, that is kind of what happened. The stool wouldn't move through normally and would sit in his intestines and get rancid.

Even now if I go in a public bathroom and the smell knocks me over I think, "Someone needs to be gluten-free!" We have been told that bowel movements are really stinky but I have found that once foods that people aren't digesting well are eliminated, stools have a relatively unoffensive smell. Not totally smell free of course, but not overwhelming either. Once those foods are eliminated, then gas also becomes less of a problem.

My son has been gluten-free since he was 18 months and about 6 years ago we realized that my husband also needed to be gluten-free due to his Crohn's disease. I agreed to go gluten-free as well to encourage my husband, and to make meal prep easier by keeping my kitchen completely gluten-free. I figured if I had gluten occasionally while I was out, it wouldn't be a big deal, but that I would generally follow a gluten-free diet as well.

Over the next few months, I had gluten occasionally. Once I ordered a grilled chicken salad and the chicken came fried. I didn't want to make more work for our waitress and figured it wasn't a big deal, so I ate it. That afternoon I got my first migraine in months. I have had migraines since childhood and realized that it has been quite a while since I had had one but didn't think too much more of it.

Over the next year or two, I would occasionally get something with gluten and would inevitably get a migraine. It became undeniable that I was reacting to gluten. Now, 6 years later, I am very sensitive to gluten and it is very obvious if I get "glutened", I get a rash on my upper arms. I had this as a child but thought everyone had it. I also get migraines, diarrhea and stomach upset that lasts for days followed by constipation when I get glutened. Thankfully, we're super careful with my son and he has rarely had a gluten reaction but my experience has helped me to know what to look for.

One grain of gluten can cause an inflammatory reaction that lasts for up to 6 months! I have learned that I need to be just as careful when ordering food out for myself as I am for my son.

Celiac and gluten intolerance often run in families. If you have family members who have had a diagnosis of IBS, Crohn's, IBD, Migraines, colon cancer or other gastrointestinal issues, and your child has gastrointestinal issues, it is a really good idea to get your child tested for Celiac. If your child tests positive or improves on a gluten-free diet, your entire family should be tested as there is a strong hereditary component to Celiac and Non-Celiac Gluten Sensitivity.

Ask your child's pediatrician or pediatric Gastroenterologist to test your child for Celiac disease if you suspect this might be an issue for your child. The doctor should run a blood test first to see if your child has the markers for Celiac disease.   A blood test for Celiac isn't 100% definitive. It can not rule out Celiac.

If the blood test comes back negative, the doctor needs to do a biopsy on the intestine to look for Celiac damage to be able to diagnose or rule out Celiac Disease.

To get correct results for Celiac tests, your child needs to be eating gluten. This is called a Gluten Challenge.   If your child is not eating gluten, then you will not get reliable results for Celiac tests as the blood test is testing for antibodies to gluten.

If your child has been doing well on a gluten-free diet and you have them go back to a gluten-containing diet for testing, your child's symptoms will return and not always leave after going gluten-free again after the tests.   It is a real risk to add back in gluten after being gluten-free. You need to discuss this with your doctor and decide if it is necessary to run the test if your child is doing well gluten-free.

Even if your child's test all come back negative for Celiac, your child might have Non-Celiac-Gluten Sensitivity. Gluten intolerance can be just as serious and just as damaging to your child as Celiac Disease.   There are no tests you can do for Non-Celiac-Gluten Sensitivity, unfortunately.

The only way to know if this is an issue for your child is to do an elimination diet.

To do an elimination diet for gluten, you need to strictly remove all gluten from your child's diet for a minimum of 30 days. It can take 4-6 months to see real improvement on a gluten-free diet but if you remove gluten for 30-60 days and then reintroduce gluten, it usually becomes very obvious if gluten is a problem.

You may not realize how much your child has improved on a gluten-free diet until you add gluten back in. My Mother-in-Law has Rheumatoid Arthritis and did a gluten-free trial. She didn't think it was making much of a difference until she ate gluten and her inflammation in her joints quickly and obviously came back even worse than before.

It can be very tricky at the beginning of a gluten-free diet to know what is safe and what is not. You must read all labels, on food, supplements, and beauty products.

Thankfully, nowadays, many products are labeled gluten-free in grocery stores. Pizza, pasta, breaded chicken nuggets, bread, rolls, pretzels, cake, donuts, and baked goods all contain gluten unless specifically made with gluten-free flour. Often there is a section in your local grocery store with gluten-free products. My son and husband both react to oats, even gluten-free certified oats. So even though a product is labeled gluten-free, I still have to read all labels to make sure it is safe for them.

We also avoid Maltodextrin which is a common ingredient in many gluten-free foods. It is a filler and a thickener and an indigestible fiber. Some maltodextrin is made with wheat, but even if it is made with corn or tapioca, it can cause gas, bloating and pain for some people with Celiac or Non-Celiac-Gluten Sensitivity or other gut health issues. It is important to avoid maltodextrin because it is highly processed, can spike blood sugar, can suppress the growth of gut bacteria, and is often made with GMO ingredients. Beyond food, maltodextrin is commonly found in supplements and probiotics so you need to read those labels too.

Many gluten-free versions of gluten-containing foods are highly processed and contain a lot of starch. This can cause blood sugar issues in many people and the lack of fiber isn't great for children struggling with constipation. For small children, using gluten-free versions of their regular food is often the easiest way to transition them to a gluten-free diet.

If your child has a self-restricted diet and the vast majority of the few things they eat contain gluten, it can feel completely overwhelming and impossible to even attempt a gluten-free diet. Often when a child has a severely limited diet, the few foods they will eat are ones they are in-tolerant of.

Gluten can work on a child's opiate receptors making them crave it like they are addicted to the few foods they will eat. If your child only eats chicken nuggets, pizza, or pasta, for exam-ple, this "addiction" to gluten can be what is causing their restricted diet. And since these foods are low in nutrition and fiber, it can lead to constipation. Once you get your child on a gluten-free diet, they will often branch out and eat a more varied diet and be willing to try new, healthier foods.

If your child will not eat gluten-free versions of their favorite foods, you can try to just feed them the foods that they will eat that do not contain gluten. Even if that severely limits the variety of foods they eat, they will not get a nutritional de-ficiency in this short period of time, especially if you are giving them a high-quality multi-vitamin.

Once your child has been off of gluten for a week or two, try a gluten-free version of one of their favorite foods. They may be willing to ac-cept it after having not eaten their "regular" food for a couple of weeks. As someone who has been gluten free for 6 years, I know that there are foods that I didn't think were very good when I first went gluten-free that I now enjoy. When you haven't had a "real" pizza for a while, a gluten-free pizza is pretty darn good but if you ate a "real" pizza yesterday then a gluten-free one is probably going to be a disappointment!

When you are newly gluten-free, it is important to be super strict to make sure you allow your child's gut to heal from the damage done by gluten. If you are ordering your child french fries, make sure the restaurant has a dedicated fryer. That means that they only fry french fries and not onion rings or chicken nuggets so you don't accidentally get any gluten on your child's fries. If there isn't a gluten-free menu, you need to ask questions of your wait staff or the chef to make sure that what you are ordering is actually safe.

Some soups are thickened with flour, some french fries are coated in wheat flour or a batter. If you order a salad you need to clarify that you can't have croutons on it and that they can't just take the croutons off of a salad, the salad needs to be made from scratch. If you order gluten free pasta for your child you need to make sure that the chef is going to boil the pasta in a pot of clean dedicated gluten-free pasta water instead of boiling gluten-free pasta in water that has been used to boil regular pasta. (Yes, this happens!) Unless the restaurant staff is properly trained in how to safely prepare gluten-free food, you need to speak up and ask questions.

As overwhelming as it can feel in the beginning to remove gluten from your child's diet, the benefits are so worth it. When you remove gluten, you have to make better choices about what foods to eat because donuts, bagels and other foods that are just carbs with very little nutrition are no longer options.

Being aware of the food that our child eats can make us more careful with our choices. I thought we had a healthy diet before my son was diagnosed with Celiac, but the diagnosis really helped change how I shopped, cooked and what I fed my family. I know my family is healthier now than they were before my son's diagnosis.

Dairy - Another Common Constipation Trigger

Dairy is a common cause of constipation. Removing dairy products, especially milk, often resolves chronic constipation in children and in adults.

A <u>Double Blind Crossover study</u>[2] was done with 65 children struggling with Chronic Constipation to see if Cow's Milk Protein was causing their constipation. Half of the children were given cow's milk for the first two weeks and the other half were given soy milk for the first two weeks without being told which one they were getting.

They all then had two weeks of being soy milk and cow's milk free, followed by two weeks where the children who were originally given cow's milk were switched to soy and the children who were given soy were switched to cow's milk. Constipation resolved for 68% of the children drinking soy milk, but none of the children drinking cow's milk.

---

[2]https://www.ncbi.nlm.nih.gov/pmc/articles/PMC3571647/

We are the only species of mammals who drink milk after the age of weaning and the only species who drink another species milk at all. Cow's milk has three times the amount of protein that human milk has and homogenization and pasteurization have made it harder for humans to be able to break down and digest the proteins because the proteins are denatured. Homogenization and pasteurization also destroy many of the enzymes that we need for digestion.

If you are past the age of one, then you don't need milk in your diet.

Beyond constipation, other signs of dairy intolerance are bloating, abdominal cramping, gas, fat in the stool, acne, seasonal allergies or congestion, and skin rashes or eczema. If you are struggling with constipation and other symptoms of dairy intolerance, I recommend strictly eliminating all dairy for at least 60 days.

You might want to request your doctor test you or your child to see if you have an allergy to dairy/Casein (the protein in milk that most people are sensitive to) before removing it from your diet. This can be necessary if your child's school requires a doctor's note to allow your child to be dairy free or for your peace of mind to know if you can attempt to add dairy back into your diet or not.

If you are concerned about getting enough Calcium and Vitamin D if you go dairy-free, many milk substitutes are fortified with calcium and Vitamin D. Leafy Greens such as spinach, kale, and collard greens or veggies like sugar snap peas or acorn squash are all great sources of calcium. Ideally, you will get Vitamin D from the sun or in a supplement along with K2.

Dairy is also very inflammatory. If you are dealing with inflammatory issues like colitis, IBS, arthritis or auto-immune diseases, going dairy free might help you.

My son and husband both have issues with dairy. Neither of them can drink milk and have no desire to, but both can tolerate some cheeses so they can have mozzarella on their gluten-free pizza for example. They both do better with hard cheeses or goat cheese in general but it is nice to have some mozzarella on occasion!

Sometimes people who react to milk can tolerate cheese, fermented organic yogurt, or Kefir. I suggest strictly removing all dairy for 60-90 days and then gradually re-introduce it to see what if any, you can tolerate. Hard aged cheeses such as sharp cheddar and parmesan are sometimes the first things that can be tolerated. But cheeses, in general, are constipating so I would be cautious and not add them back in until you have your constipation under control.

Using lactose-free milk will not help end your constipation. Lactose is a sugar. Casein is the protein that is causing constipation.

If you want to try non-dairy alternatives like Almond Milk, Flax Milk, Pea Protein Milk, or Coconut Milk, make sure to look for ones that do not have Carrageenan in them. Carrageenan is made from seaweed and is marketed as a natural additive but it is very damaging to the gut and can cause a lot of problems for people with gut issues. I would also only use organic versions of alternative kinds of milk. Look for versions with the least amount of ingredients.

It is challenging to go dairy free but it is worth it if it ends your child's struggle with constipation permanently.

Hypothyroidism and Childhood Constipation

One of the least talked about symptoms of hypothyroidism is constipation but it is a very common symptom. In fact, Constipation can be the only symptom of hypothyroidism.

If your child is suffering from constipation and doctors haven't been able to figure out why, it could be due to hypothyroidism. If your child has hypothyroidism and is on medication for it, constipation is often a sign that he or she is being under-dosed even if their lab values are "In Range."

Because children aren't expected to have hypothyroidism, it can be something that doctors don't even look for when you bring your child in for constipation.

Beyond constipation, other signs of hypothyroidism include: weight gain; fatigue; dry skin; puffy face; muscle weakness; aches; tenderness; joint pain; stiffness or swelling; irregular menstrual periods; dry hair or hair loss; increased sensitivity to cold; and highblood cholesterol levels. In children, undiagnosed or under-treated hypothyroidism can also lead to delayed or poor growth and delayed puberty or precocious puberty. Hypothyroidism is especially common in children with Down's Syndrome or diabetes.

Hypothyroidism slows the metabolism of your body which slows the action of the digestive system. This causes stool to be in the intestines and colon longer. The longer stool is in the digestive system, the more water gets pulled out of the stool. The stool gets larger and harder to pass.

Hypothyroidism also weakens the contractions of the muscles needed to push through the stool so it is harder to push the poop out. This can make very painful, hard to pass stools. In children, this can lead to withholding of the stool due to fear of passing a painful stool.

All too often, physicians only test TSH when looking for thyroid problems. TSH stands for Thyroid Stimulating Hormone. It isn't even a thyroid hormone but a pituitary hormone that signals the thyroid to put out thyroid hormones. There is also a large range that many doctors feel is acceptable for TSH but if your child is in the upper end of that range they can feel horrible and be constipated.

Ideally, you will find a physician who is willing to run a full thyroid panel. If you can not find a doctor willing to run a full thyroid panel, I have resources for lab testing on my website.

https://naturalconstipationsolutions.com/recommended-lab-testing-for-chronic-constipation/

Once you get their full thyroid panel results you want to look and see if your child's results are not just in range but Optimal. Your full panel should include TSH, Free T3, Free T4, Reverse T3 and thyroid antibodies.

It can be hard to get endocrinologists, pediatricians or family care doctors to help you get your child's levels to the optimal range. If they are being treated with just T4 medications, then it can be even more challenging to get to an optimal range and standard doctors often only prescribe T4 (Levothyroxine, Synthroid). T4 is a synthetic hormone.

Using a Natural Desiccated Thyroid (NDT) medication like Armour or Nature-Thyroid, instead of a T4 medication often helps with constipation and other hypothyroid symptoms. NDT's contain complete dried thyroid glands of pigs or cows so it contains all of the thyroid hormones, T4, T3, T2 and other elements that are in a thyroid gland and that your child's thyroid gland may not be making, or have the ability to convert to the hormones they need.

T4 is a storage hormone. In theory, when your child is dosed with T4, their body will convert it to the active hormone, T3. Unfortunately, if their thyroid gland isn't working properly, then it may not convert the T4 to T3 properly. They can not have enough T3, which causes hypo symptoms like constipation, and also high levels of Reverse T3 (an inactive form of T3).

If your child has high Reverse T3, it acts like a brake on their metabolism. This can lead to constipation and weight gain. High Reverse T3, also called Pooling, can be treated by using T3 (Cytomel) medication. High levels of Reverse T3 can be caused by very low calorie diets, chronic illness or infections, chronic inflammation, chronic untreated gut infections or imbalance, chronic emotional stressors, and certain medications like antidepressants, narcotics, anti-seizure meds, blood pressure meds and diabetic medications.

Another level that must be tested is thyroid antibodies. Over 90% of cases of hypothyroidism are due to Hashimoto's Disease, an autoimmune disease. Anti-thyroperoxidase (anti-TPO) and anti-thyroglobulin (TgAb) are elevated in autoimmune hypothyroidism. Both Anti-TPO and TgAb need to be tested, not just one or the other. If your child has these antibodies, they have Hashimoto's. Some experts believe that any thyroid antibodies, even if they don't reach the abnormal range, is a sign of having Hashimoto's Disease.

If tests show any thyroid antibodies, you need to keep a close eye on the levels and do what you can to bring them down. One of the most important things you can do to lower your child's antibodies is going gluten and dairy free.

The proteins in gluten and dairy can cause inflammation in the thyroid gland and trigger the production of antibodies. Any autoimmune disease benefits from a gluten free and dairy free diet. Gluten and dairy are two of the main triggers in constipation so removing them can also be hugely beneficial for constipation.

Often, going gluten and dairy free is enough to lower Hashimoto's antibodies and no other treatments are needed. It is often necessary to also avoid soy (especially non-organic and non-fermented soy) and eggs if your child has Hashimoto's.

Supplementing with Vitamin A is also something to consider if you are struggling with hypothyroidism. When our thyroid isn't functioning properly, we can't get enough Vitamin A. Our thyroid is responsible for the conversion of beta-carotene to Vitamin A. If your thyroid is low, then you won't convert enough. Also, if you are deficient in Vitamin A, it can lead to hypothyroidism, so it works both ways. Low Vitamin A is a common reason why patients don't respond to thyroid hormone supplementation.

Vitamin A RDA:
6-12 months 350 mcg
1-6 years 400 mcg
7-10 years 500 mcg
11-14 600 mcg
15 and older males 700 mcg and 15 and older females 600 mcg

Low Vitamin D can make you susceptible to developing Hashimoto's Disease and can increase TPO antibody production. To properly metabolize Vitamin D, supplementing with Vitamin K at the same time is recommended.

The RDA for Vitamin D:
Infants 10 mcg
Children, teens and adults 15 mcg daily

When you supplement with Vitamins A, D and K you can decrease your TSH by up to 33%, increase your active hormone T3 by up to 61% and reduce TPO antibodies by up to 46% (Forefronthealth.com)

Often, once you get your child properly medicated, their diet adjusted to bring down their antibodies, and the proper supplements are introduced into their regiment, the child's constipation resolves without any other interventions being needed.

The Importance of Gut Bacteria

Our modern sanitary lifestyles, with processed foods, antibacterial soaps, living in air-conditioned homes and driving to our air-conditioned schools and offices in our air-conditioned cars, glyphosate, rounds of antibiotics for sickness, and antibiotics in our meat and dairy products, have led us to an epidemic of constipation due to a lack of good healthy bacteria in our digestive system.

We need healthy gut flora and when they are killed off, there are serious consequences for our health. Good gut bacteria plays many necessary roles in our bodies including helping us break down our food, getting the benefit from the vitamins, minerals, and nutrients in our food, makes nutrients we can't make on our own and even communication with the cells in our bodies.

Probiotics are great for short-term use after a viral infection or after an antibiotic or when you are trying to get bacteria in your very picky child and they refuse fermented foods but even the best probiotics used long-term can cause you to develop a monoculture of bacteria.

When you look at a bottle of probiotics, it will state how many billion live cultures it contains. This sounds very impressive. But the truth is that these are just billions of copies of a very limited number of bacteria. Most probiotics contain 1-13 strains of bacteria and those few strains are multiplied over and over again until you get X Billion copies of the same strain.

When you make wild fermented foods and drinks, you get trillions of wild bacteria from the air and you get more variety of types of bacteria than you will ever get from a store-bought probiotic. Plus, wild lacto-fermented foods and drinks are significantly cheaper than high quality probiotics.

But I know that it isn't always possible, or practical, to rely on just fermented foods and drinks for gut bacteria. Adding in a rotation of high-quality probiotics can make a huge difference in gut health. I recommend rotating probiotics to a new brand with different strains after each bottle is done.

Our guts are meant to have tens of thousands of different strains of bacteria and when you use the same probiotic with just a few limited strains of bacteria for long periods of time, you end up populating your gut with millions of copies of just a few strains of bacteria. Having a few strains of good bacteria is so much better than no good bacteria, because you then your gut gets overrun with bad bacteria, but it still isn't the best solution.

Make sure that the next bottle of probiotic has different strains than the previous bottle so you are introducing the most variety of bacteria possible into your child's gut.

It can be hard to convince your child to eat or drink fermented foods. Although I will also say that many people figure their kids will never eat anything fermented so they don't even try.
You might be surprised! My son is relatively picky when it comes to the taste and texture of foods. He doesn't love every fermented food I make, but he adores my fermented carrots and pickles. He thinks that fermented carrots are a huge treat and he loves his "probiotic lemonade."

Another great way to get beneficial bacteria into your child's intestines is to go to different locations and breathe different air. Traveling to the beach, the mountains, the desert, National Parks, the lake, the mountains and anywhere in between, is a good way to expand your gut bacteria.

Plant a garden and then encourage your kids to play in the dirt with you, help you weed, pick cherry tomatoes off of the vine and eat them without washing them. Even if you live in an apartment you can grow herbs or a cherry tomato plant on your balcony or in a window. Take your kids to the park and let them play in the sandbox. Let them run on the grass with bare feet and breath in diverse bacteria in the air and from the soil.

Lastly, before we start talking about specific probiotics, please throw out your antibacterial soaps! Use Castile soap or another natural soap that doesn't contain triclosan or other antibacterial agents.

Also, avoid toothpaste that contains PEG/Polyethylene Glycol. It is important to read all of the labels on your personal care products to ensure they they don't contain PEG or antibacterial ingredients. Otherwise, they will undo the good work you are doing repopulating your child's gut bacteria.

PEG kills off bacteria in the gut so if your child has been on Miralax, they really need their gut bacteria repopulated.

I learned how damaging PEG is when my son was prescribed Miralax at age 4. He was diagnosed with Megacolon and the pediatric Gastro told me that he would need Miralax for life to be able to have normal bowel movements. During the time my son was on Miralax, his health went downhill. He developed tics, anxiety, panic attacks, OCD and was eventually diagnosed with autism.

I have spent the last few years working to heal the damage that Miralax caused. One of the biggest things we have done to heal his gut is to work on rebuilding gut bacteria. I'm really lucky that he loves fermented carrots, fermented pickles and a few other fermented foods. We do use probiotics here and there, especially if we travel, or if he's sick.

When you are looking for a high-quality probiotic you want to look for one with a variety of strains of bacteria. If there is just one, it might help briefly but it isn't going to make a huge difference long-term in your child's struggle with constipation.

Unfortunately, high-quality probiotics are expensive. If you are getting a cheap probiotic, there are no guarantees that the bacteria is alive or will survive the stomach acid. Look for probiotics that need to be refrigerated. If you are ordering them during the summer months, then make sure they are being shipped in a cooler with ice packs. If you are buying them locally, look for a store that keeps probiotics in a refrigerator.

Some people find that when they introduce probiotics they can develop gas. When you give probiotics to your child I would start low and slow and build up the dose over time watching for any issues they might have.

Many probiotics are dairy based. If your child is sensitive to dairy, it is something to look at. Even people who can't eat or drink dairy can often tolerate dairy based probiotics. The only way to know is to try.

When we have to use a probiotic, we usually use Visbiome. It comes in pills and sachets. You can mix the powder from the sachet into cold food for your child if they can't or won't swallow a pill. You can also open the pills up and use the powder in the pills. Visbiome isn't dairy free but my husband, who is sensitive to dairy, has no issues with the minute amount of dairy in Visbiome and is very happy with the results.

If you are dealing with constipation with an infant, there is a wonderful option from Klaire Labs called Ther-biotic infant probiotic. Many infants are constipated because they were born by C-section and didn't receive the beneficial bacteria they would have gotten from their mother during a vaginal birth. Also, if your baby is on formula, they don't get the bacteria that they would get from their mother's milk so even if they aren't having problems digesting cow's milk or another alternative formula, they are still not getting the bacteria that they would get from breast milk.

If your baby has been on antibiotics, then adding in a high-quality probiotic can also help with repopulating their gut flora. You can mix it with formula or put some on your nipple if you are breastfeeding.

For older children aged 2 and up, Klaire Labs makes a Children's Chewable Ther-Biotic.

Most probiotics that need to be refrigerated are okay for a couple of weeks at room temperature but if it is hot out, then I would try to find it locally or order a different probiotic that is shipped in a cooler with ice packs.

If you are looking for a powder probiotic, Klaire Labs Ther-biotic Complete Powder is a good option. You can sprinkle it on food or mix it with cold drinks or soft foods. This is an adult formula but it says to discuss dosing with your child's physician.   Depending on the age and weight and gut health of your child, you might be able to adjust the dose based on the amount of probiotics in an adult dose.

Garden of Life Raw Probiotics are shipped cold from Amazon and many members of my Facebook group, Natural Constipation Solutions, have reported excellent success with them. This probiotic also contains Inulin, which is a prebiotic fiber. For some children, it can worsen constipation and for some, it improves it. Keep an eye on your child if you are trying it. This probiotic is safe for infants 3 months and up so it is a good option for infants who were born by C-section, are bottle fed or have been on antibiotics.

If you are interested in trying an easy, child-friendly ferment, the recipe below is a fun place to start. It won't work with every probiotic discussed above, such as chewables or gummies, but if you have powder, capsules or sachets of probiotic, then you can use the probiotic as a starter in this and other fermentation recipes.

You can make this fermented lemonade with lemons or limes and then blend it with a tray of ice. It is a great way to get lots of fluids into your child, since dehydration can be a contributing factor in constipation. I have found that just making a slushee is a great way to get your child to drink a lot of fluid without any fight. This has the added advantage of furnishing lots of good bacteria, too!

Fermented Lemonade Made with Probiotics
2 liters of water
1 organic lemon's juice
1-4 capsules of probiotic
1-2 Tbs organic sugar

Add 2 liters of water to a container. Add lemon juice, probiotic and sugar. Stir until sugar is dissolved. Cover loosely with a cloth or coffee filter. Steep overnight on the counter and then put it in the fridge until it is cold or serve over ice.

Once you experiment with fermented foods and drinks and see how easy and inexpensive it is, I hope it empowers you to add more ferments to your diet. Many grocery stores and health food stores are also now selling lacto-fermented pickles and drinks that are also good options and an easy way to try different fermented to see what your child will enjoy.

Working on improving the variety of bacteria in your child's gut can go a long way towards helping them in their struggle with chronic constipation.

Fiber and Constipation

Often when we take our kids into the pediatrician and explain that our child is constipated, the doctor tells us to increase fiber as a solution. While so much better advice than prescribing a laxative like Miralax, fiber can actually worsen constipation in some cases.

I polled my readers and asked if adding fiber supplements helped their child's constipation or worsened it. I suspected that fiber would make it worse in a percentage of children but was honestly surprised that well over 50% of the respondents reported that fiber made their child's constipation worse. But the parents who reported that it helped their child, said that adding fiber made a huge difference with their child and helped them so much. So we need to look closely at fiber, how it works in the digestive system and evaluate whether you should try it with your child.

There are two types of fiber; soluble and insoluble. Soluble fiber draws in water to the stool and makes the stool softer and easier to pass. Insoluble fiber bulks up the stool and can help it pass through the intestines. Fruits, veggies, nuts, and seeds are all great sources of both soluble and insoluble fiber. But it can be tricky to get enough fiber in your child through diet. Especially if you have a child with autism or sensory issues that self restrict their diet to foods like white bread (.5-1 grams of fiber), chicken nuggets (1 gram) and pizza (2.5 grams of fiber) Raw and cooked vegetables have a similar amount of fiber but cooking makes the cellulose softer, making it easier to digest for some people.

Amount of fiber your child needs:

1-3	19 grams of fiber
4-8	25 grams of fiber
9-13	Boys 31 grams and girls 26 grams
14-19	Boys 38 grams and girls 26 grams

It can be tricky, especially with a less than ideal diet, to get enough dietary fiber in your child to prevent constipation. A half cup of cooked veggies have 2-4 grams and a small piece of fruit has about 3 grams of fiber. If you are gluten-free, most gluten-free baked goods are lower in fiber than the wheat flour versions because gluten-free flours are often filled with starches which are low in fiber.

Fiber supplements are one option to get more fiber in your child.

SmartyPants Complete Vitamin with Fiber are a good option if you want to try a supplement. A 4 gummie serving has 4 grams of soluble prebiotic fiber. Prebiotic fiber feeds gut bacteria so having prebiotic fiber is very important. My son is very picky with supplements but he liked the flavor and texture of these gummies.

I like the Smarty Pants brand of vitamins because they are non-GMO and use high-quality natural ingredients like turmeric and black carrot juice for coloring. They use Chickory Root for the Inulin Fiber. Inulin also increases Butyrate in the gut which helps with constipation.

When trying to add a fiber supplement like Smarty Pants you need to make sure you get your child drinking a lot. If they are dehydrated then the fiber will not have enough fluid and will make the stool dry and hard to pass.

Culturelle Probiotics with Fiber contain 3.5 grams of fiber plus prebiotic inulin and is gluten free and dairy free. Adding probiotics is always a good option when you are dealing with constipation.

A fun, kid-friendly food option to add fiber is the Mama Chia Fruit and Chia Pouches. They have 7 grams of fiber and come in kid-friendly flavors and pouches so you can send them in lunches.

When doing your grocery shopping you can also look for better choices to buy, whole grains instead of white options. Choose brown rice over white rice for example. Brown Rice has 1.1 grams of fiber in 1/3 cup versus just .2 grams for white rice. White rice has had the husk, bran, and germ removed and that is where all of the fiber is. Instead of making a peanut butter sandwich, serve your child peanut butter on celery or with whole grain crackers.

If you are gluten free, many gluten-free options are very low in fibers. Look for gluten-free options that use seeds, whole grain flours or whole seed flours instead of starch or white rice flour.

Juice has had most of the fiber stripped away and is mostly sugar. The whole fruit or veggie is always a better choice than the juiced version. If you have ever used a juicer you know that there is a ton of fiber that is left at the end of making juice.

Some kids just do not do well with fiber supplements or even high fiber diets. If you add any of these supplements or foods and notice an increase of constipation, even with adequate hydration, then you might want to investigate if your child has motility issues or low tone. If you suspect motility issues, ask your child's doctor to do a motility study on your child. You might also want to try a low fiber diet for a period of time and see if it helps your child's constipation.

Fiber is definitely not a "one size fits everyone" solution. If your child can't tolerate fiber now, take a break and try it again when you are further along in your gut healing protocol.

I always prefer to give my child nutrition through real food instead of supplements if at all possible. Start reading labels and see if you can increase the fiber in your child's diet by picking higher fiber options.

Flaxseeds are a good source of fiber. Whole flaxseed has 3 grams of fiber per Tablespoon and 2.2 grams of fiber if it is ground. Flaxseed is high in Omega 3 fatty acids. Omega 3 Fatty acids can cause diarrhea in some people so increasing your intake of fatty acids is helpful for some people with constipation. It is also believed that flaxseed speeds up the movement in the intestines, moving food through the gut faster, reducing constipation.

Flaxseed goes rancid quickly so should be stored in the refrigerator. Whole flaxseed can be stored for a year but ground goes badly much more quickly. You want to use ground flaxseed to get the full benefit of the nutrients. I recommend grinding whole flaxseed just before you use it. You can add ground flaxseed to smoothies, yogurt, applesauce, recipes for baked goods or even in meatloaf or hamburger patties.

One of my favorite ways to get easily digestible fiber in my child's diet is with chia seeds. Chia seeds have 11 grams of fiber in just two Table-spoons! 2 tbs also contains 30% of your RDA of magnesium and a great ratio of Omega 3 to Omega 6 fatty acids. They have been used since Mayan times when Mayan warriors ate them for strength and endurance.

Chia seeds are also very high in magnesium, 80mg in 2 Tbs. Magnesium is a critical mineral for constipation relief and most of our kids are deficient in it.

When introducing chia seeds to the diet, start slowly until you know how your child will handle them. In some, they can increase constipation and bloating. If this happens to your child, I would work on healing their gut and I would add probiotics before trying to add fiber again.

Chia seeds swell when soaked in liquid. You want to soak them for 15 minutes minimum to make sure they have absorbed as much fluid as possible before ingesting them. If they soak up fluid in your intestines they can make the stool dry and hard to pass. So make sure they are hydrated before you consume them.

Chia seeds are super versatile. My first experi-ence with chia seeds came as a substitution for eggs when my son was young and couldn't tolerate eggs, even in baked goods. I would make a "chia egg" and add it to pancakes, bread or anything else that needed an egg.

To make a chia egg you are going to need to grind up the chia seeds. I use a coffee grinder that is used exclusively for grinding seeds and herbs, otherwise your chia will taste like coffee. Grind just over 1 Tbs of chia seeds in your grinder (you will get close to 2 Tbs of ground) then measure out 1 Tbs of chia and add 3 Tbs of water. Mix well and put in the fridge for 15 minutes while it sets up. Then you can add it to your baking instead of eggs.

Even if your child can eat eggs, this substitution is a great way to increase the fiber in your child's favorite baked goods. This is a wonderful option if your child has sensory issues with food because the chia seeds are ground up and relatively unobtrusive in their food.

You can sprinkle chia seeds in smoothies, add to baked goods, make a "boba tea" kind of drink that has a super silly texture, make a chia seed jam with fresh fruit, add to breading for fish or chicken, sprinkle them on yogurt, cereal or oatmeal or on your salad or cut up fruit or mix into dips, guacamole or hummus.

It may take some experimenting to find out if fiber helps your child's constipation or worsens it and if it helps it, how much to use for the best results. If your child can't tolerate fiber at all, work on healing your child's gut and getting their constipation under control by other means and then try to reintroduce fiber again down the road.

Low Tone or Hypotonia as a Cause of Chronic Constipation

Low Tone or Hypotonia means that your child has low muscle tone. The Occupational Therapist who diagnosed my son quizzed me on things like how old my son was when he started to crawl and how did he crawl. Was it a traditional crawl, army crawl etc.

My son had a unique crawl that his older brother and my mom all did. They sat up with one leg in front and pulled the other leg through. My grandma laughed when she saw my kids crawl because it brought back happy memories of my mom crawling the exact same way.

Unfortunately, that crawl was a sign of low tone. Their core wasn't strong enough to allow them to do the traditional crawl.

Articulation issues with speech, delayed turning over, delayed crawling and walking, poor posture, fatiguing quickly, increased flexibility and delays with gross motor skills are all signs of low tone.

When your child has low tone, the muscles that help push out the stool don't work as well as they should. The stool stays in the intestines longer and dries out, making it bulkier and harder to push out. Your child can also be pushing as hard as they can but because the muscles aren't strong enough to move the stool through, the child has a hard time getting the stool to come out.

The OT had us work on exercises to increase my son's core strength. One of the exercises was having my son relearn to crawl, even though he was 6 years old. The OT threw down a ton of regular bed pillows on the floor and had my son crawl across them to get a toy on the other side. Our insurance didn't cover OT and it cost us $250 for my son to crawl across those pillows.

You can buy some pillows for cheap and still be less than half of the cost of a single OT session! And your child can use them over and over. You can do different games with your child and the pillows. Time them and see if they can beat their time. Have them race across, retrieve something and bring it to you or just let them play on them. Even sitting on them, with them being uneven and soft, will force your child to do tiny core corrections that will help to build up core muscles.

The OT at our local school had some great recommendations for us to work on low tone. She suggested buying a bean bag chair. She sug-

gested that he sit in it to do his school work instead of sitting at a table or desk. My son loves
the chair. It also helps by giving a "hug" of deep
pressure which can be super comforting to kids
with sensory issues.

She also suggested that we get my son a swing
for my son's room. We picked out a hammock
swing chair for my son. He loves the cocoon
feeling of being inside of it. It takes a lot of work
for him to get it to swing back and forth which
helps him build core strength. He stands in the
swing and can get it going pretty fast or he sits
in the swing and pushes off the walls to make it
swing. This involves him bending forward and
using all of his tummy muscles to push off. But
he can also sit in it and read a book and chill
with his cat!

If you can't install it because you live in an
apartment or you don't want to install it from
your ceiling, then look for a swing that hangs
from a bar that fits in your doorway. It fits over
your door like a pull-up bar so it doesn't cause
any damage and it is very strong.

All of this equipment will help your child to build
up core strength and it is less than one OT session. We have a swing outside but the one in my
son's room is used way more and is a great way
to get energy out on cold or rainy or too hot to
play outside days.

One of the best recommendations from the school OT was to buy my son a mini trampoline and keep it in our living room. It isn't the most attractive decoration to have in your living room and we regularly are walking around it as it is often in our way, but it has made the biggest difference in my son's constipation. We often joke that he bounces down the poop. Often after bouncing for a few minutes, he HAS to go.

Beyond bouncing, you can work with your child on the trampoline to build core strength by standing on one foot and stretching their arms out. Have them move their arms like a clock. If you are working on how to tell time, you can shout out times and have them try to do the times with their arms. Have them bounce on one foot and then on the other. Many kids with low tone favor one side over the other so working on both is important.

Drop toys or coins on the trampoline. Then challenge them to stand on one foot, bend over and pick them up one at a time. Invent fun games for them to play on the trampoline.

My son and I love to hike in the woods. Walking, especially over uneven ground, up and down hills and jumping over creeks, is a great way to build core strength. Often after a hike, he will have a bowel movement within an hour or two of coming home. This is free, fun and you are building memories as well and getting in shape.

We are lucky to live within walking distance of a wildlife management area with a trail down to a lake. It takes us about an hour to do the round trip to the lake and back. And it is all uphill ALL the way home, which really works the core muscles. You can add in a silly walk competition, suggest picking up sticks or rocks in the path or march like soldiers to add to core strength building and make the walk extra productive.

I also signed my son up for therapeutic horseback riding lessons a few years ago. Horseback riding is an excellent way to work on core strength. It has also been amazing for my son's anxiety and has helped him in so many ways. He has been riding for over 3 years and it has been a wonderful experience for him. If you are working with a therapeutic stable, they will understand low tone and help him to work on core strength but any horseback riding lessons will help. Our farm works with very young and special needs children. He's gotten more out of it than OT and it is less expensive.

Swimming is another great way to build core strength. We don't have a pool but have a friend who does. We also plan vacations where there are hotel pools! Aquatots offers indoor swimming lessons for little ones or check out your local Y.

A simple way to increase core strength is using either a Balance Ball chair or a Wobble

Cushion. Your child sitting on a balance ball chair or Wobble cushion will make them constantly correct their posture working the muscles in their core. I bought 2 of the Wobble cushions and put one on my son's dining room chair and one on the floor under his feet. My older son tried them and loved them so much he wanted me to get them for him too. Your child can also stand on the Wobble cushion to build strength. My next purchase is the Balance Ball Chair. Our Integrative Medicine physician has them in his office and my son is obsessed.

Helping my son build his core strength has really helped him with his constipation and his ability to push out his stool.

Tests to Run to Help You Get to the Root Cause of Your Child's Chronic Constipation

To solve your constipation or your child's constipation, you need to figure out what is causing constipation in the first place. There are tests that can be run that will help you to figure out what is the root cause of chronic or functional constipation.

X-RAY

X-ray of a
Constipated Child

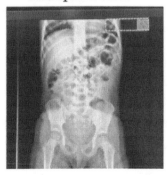

X-ray of child
after cleanout

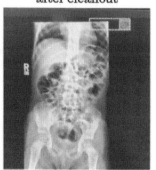

The first test most doctors run for constipation is an X-ray. If you are unsure if you or your child is constipated or if you are concerned about a blockage, ask your doctor to do an X-ray to see what kind of back up or blockage you are dealing with. Often a second X-ray is done after doing a clean-out to make sure that the clean-out was effective.

There are concerns from having too many X-rays run due to radiation so I would be cautious about having multiple X-rays done for constipation.

ANORECTAL MANOMETRY

Anorectal manometry uses a catheter and a balloon to look at the nerves and muscles of the anus and rectum. It tests sensations and pressure in the anus and rectum. The catheter is attached to a computer that records the pressure. Anorectal manometry tests whether children have normal sensation and are using their muscles correctly to hold and pass stool. It also helps to diagnose a condition called Hirschsprung disease and congenital megacolon.

If your child is a chronic withholder, this is a test to request because they might have muscles that contract instead of push, causing them to appear to withhold when they are not able to properly push out their stool. This will also help determine if your child gets the sensation to push which many children with chronic constipation struggle with because they either have congenital megacolon or Hirschsprung's Disease where the nerves didn't travel fully down the child's rectum during the first trimester or their colon is so stretched out from being chronically filled with stool that they lose sensation of having to go.

ENDOSCOPY

An endoscopy can show if you have Celiac. Celiac is known for causing diarrhea but it can also cause constipation. Blood tests for Celiac are not always accurate so a negative blood test does not mean that you do not have Celiac, the only way to be sure if you do or not, is through an endoscopy.

COLONOSCOPY

A colonoscopy can determine if you or your child has Crohn's disease or Ulcerative Colitis. Symptoms can include constipation, diarrhea, cramping, abdominal pain, fever, rectal bleeding.

MRI

An MRI can show if your child has a Tethered Cord.

- If your child has had constipation from birth,

- Hairy patches, dimples, fatty tumors on the lower back or lesions
- Foot deformities
- Spinal deformities
- Leg weakness
- Abnormal gait, walking on the tips of toes, wearing the tips or side of one shoe
- Low back pain
- Scoliosis
- Urinary irregularities

If you see these issues, then it is good to ask your doctor to look into tethered cord.

There are some lab tests that can help you determine the cause of your constipation. You can request that your doctor run these tests if you think they could be contributing to your constipation.

The following information on testing is taken from the testing website <u>True Health Labs.</u> You can order labs directly through them if your doctor won't order them for you.

Complete Thyroid Panel

The Complete Thyroid Test Panel reveals imbalances that are otherwise not tested in routine lab tests and helps better identify the root cause of thyroid dysfunction.

What's being tested in this panel:
- TSH
- Total T4
- Total T3
- Free T4
- Free T3
- Reverse T3 (rT3)
- T3U
- Free T4 Index
- TPO and Anti-TG Antibodies (Hashimoto's Screen, thyroid antibodies

Complete Celiac Panel

This test panel is designed to screen for a potential autoimmune attack to the lining of the gut, also known as celiac disease.

What's Being Tested:
- Endomysial Antibody IgA
- Immunoglobulin A (Total IgA)
- Tissue Transglutaminase (tTG) IgA
- Tissue Transglutaminase (tTG) IgG

Gluten Sensitivity/Celiac Disease Panel

What's Being Tested:
- Endomysial Antibody IgA

- Immunoglobulin A (Total IgA)
- Tissue Transglutaminase (IgG + IgA)
- HLA DQ2 + HLA DQ8 Genetic Test for Celiac Disease
- Gliadin Antibodies IgG + IgA

DNA Stool Test

The GI Effects Comprehensive Stool Profile can reveal important information about the root cause of many common gastrointestinal symptoms such as gas, bloating, indigestion, abdominal pain, diarrhea, and constipation. This stool analysis utilizes biomarkers such as Calprotectin to differentiate between Inflammatory Bowel Disease (IBD) and Irritable Bowel Syndrome. Genova's GI Effects test can be used to evaluate patients with a clinical history that suggests a gastrointestinal infection or dysbiosis.

Gut microbes are codependent with one another and with their human host, and the health of one affects the other. A sizeable volume of research associates a dysbiotic, or imbalanced gut microbiome with multiple diseases both within and outside of the GI tract including constipation.

Leaky Gut Test - Lactulose and Mannitol

The Leaky Gut Test (or Intestinal Permeability Test) is a noninvasive gastrointestinal test that measures small intestinal absorption and barrier function in the bowel. Malabsorption and increased intestinal permeability (leaky gut) can be associated with chronic gastrointestinal imbalances.

The Leaky Gut Test requires you take a baseline morning urine sample (done at home). Once completed, you will be required to drink a mixture of two non-metabolized sugars, **lactulose, and mannitol**. After six hours, you will collect an additional sample of urine. The lab will measure how much lactulose and mannitol was excreted.

If Leaky Gut Syndrome is NOT present, the large lactulose molecules should remain in the GI tract and thus test low in the urine. If the count is high in the urine, Leaky Gut Syndrome should be considered.

Possible Causes of Leaky Gut:
- Intestinal infection
- Ingestion of allergenic foods
- Trauma
- Toxic chemicals
- NSAIDs such as aspirin, ibuprofen, naproxen etc.
- Antibiotics

HOW CAN THE LEAKY GUT TEST HELP?

The Leaky Gut Test is extremely important when beginning restorative treatment plans. As intestinal health improves, the lactulose/mannitol ratio should improve.

WHAT'S BEING TESTED IN THIS PANEL?

- Creatine
- Lactulose
- Mannitol
- Total Urine Volume
- Includes: Mannitol/Lactulose Drink

Food Allergy Test

Your body can attack food as a foreign invader similarly to the way it attacks bacteria and viruses. Food allergy testing is used to identify foods that the immune system overreacts to. This over-reaction produces inflammation. Food allergy testing can help you remove foods that promote inflammation and help you add foods that are safe to eat. When you eliminate foods you react to, your constipation will improve.

WHAT TO DO WITH THE FOOD ALLERGY RESULTS.

Most IgG food allergies need to be avoided for 6-12 months before attempting to add them back into your diet. If you experience a recurrence of constipation, remove the food again.

OAT Test/Organic Acids

Organic acids are byproducts of our metabolism. High amounts of these organic acid byproducts can cause ill-health. Knowing which metabolic processes to improve is essential to living well and reversing chronic disease.

The Organic Acids Test (OAT) offers a comprehensive metabolic snapshot of a patient's overall health with over 70 markers. It provides an accurate evaluation of intestinal yeast and bacteria.

Abnormally high levels of these microorganisms can cause or worsen behavior disorders, hyperactivity, movement disorders, fatigue, and immune function. Many people with chronic illnesses and neurological disorders often excrete several abnormal organic acids in their urine. The cause of these high levels could include oral antibiotic use, high sugar diets, immune deficiencies, acquired infections, as well as genetic factors.

The Organic Acids Test also includes markers for vitamin and mineral levels, oxidative stress, neurotransmitter levels, and is the only OAT to include markers for oxalates, which are highly correlated with many chronic illnesses.

If abnormalities are detected using the OAT, treatments can include supplements, such as vitamins and antioxidants, or dietary modification. Upon treatment, patients and practitioners have reported significant improvement such as decreased fatigue, regular bowel function, increased energy and alertness, increased concentration, improved verbal skills, less hyperactivity, and decreased abdominal pain.

This Organix® test also looks for the metabolic byproducts of several bacteria and yeast.

If your child has been on Miralax this is an important test to run as Miralax can cause an elevation in oxalic acid. If your child developed kidney issues while on Miralax, I also recommend getting this test run.

Occult Blood Stool Test

What's Being Tested:

• **Occult Blood**

A fecal occult blood test looks at a sample of your stool (feces) to check for blood. Occult blood means that you can't see it with the naked eye. Blood in the stool means there is some kind of bleeding in the intestines. This bleeding may be caused by a variety of conditions, including:

- Polyps
- Hemorrhoids
- diverticulitis
- Ulcers
- Colitis, a type of inflammatory bowel disease

Intestinal Parasites Stool Test

Parasite infections do not just cause gastrointestinal symptoms, an increasing number of parasite cases have full-body complaints that are not traditionally associated with parasites, such as:

- Urticaria
- Reactive arthritis
- Chronic fatigue syndrome
- Asthma
- Constipation in individuals who are immune-compromised or whose intestinal flora is chronically imbalanced

Genova's Parasitology Test

Genova's Parasite test uses the most advanced procedures to identify a wide range of protozoan parasites, including amoebae, flagellates, ciliates, and microsporidia.

What's Being Tested:
- Bacteriology, aerobic x3
- Bacteriology, anaerobic
- Cryptosporidium
- Entamoeba histolytica
- Giardia lamblia
- Parasite Identification, Concentrate
- Parasite Identification,TrichromeStain
- Yeast Culture

Yeast Culture Stool Test

WHAT'S BEING TESTED:

- Yeast Culture (stool)

A Yeast Culture will help you find out if over-growth of yeast is contributing to your issues with yeast infections, gas, bloating, digestion, constipation, diarrhea, IBS. Overgrowth of yeast and fungi in the gastrointestinal tract can occur due to frequent antibiotic use, auto-immune conditions, and diets high in sugar and refined carbohydrates.

Often it is difficult to get a standard doctor or gastroenterologist to run the tests that you need run to help with constipation. I have resources on my website to help you find a functional, in-tegrative doctor or a naturopath.

Go to the link below for more information on how to find a doctor who can help you in your area.

https://naturalconstipationsolutions.com/find-a-doctor-help-root-cause-constipation/

If you can not find a doctor who will help you, then there are other options to be able to get the labs run that you need to have run. For more resources on where you can order your own tests directly without needing a doctor's pre-scription go to

https://naturalconstipationsolutions.com/rec-ommended-lab-testing-for-chronic-constipation/

Heal Your Child's Gut

Many children struggle for weeks or even years with chronic constipation. Chronic constipation can stretch out the colon and cause damage, making it hard for the child to know when they have to go. Laxatives can cause their own damage. The initial cause of the constipation such as gluten intolerance or diary intolerance, can also cause damage to the gut.

The first step to healing your child's gut is to remove processed foods made with preservatives, food colors, anything with an ingredient that has a number after it, maltodextrin, carrageenan and anything that you can't pronounce. I try to make most of our food from scratch but if I do buy pre-made foods, I try to limit them to foods with a small number of recognizable ingredients.

Switching to organic food is very important. When we buy food that isn't organic, it often has glyphosate or other herbicides and pesticides on it. We are eating a product that will kill off the bacteria in our gut. We need a large and varied number of bacteria to have good digestion. The bacteria in our gut does a lot of the work of digesting our food.

A diet like the Specific Carbohydrate Diet or the Autoimmune Protocol are excellent options to work on healing your child's gut. It is tricky to change a child's diet but it is possible. At a minimum, try an elimination diet removing gluten, dairy, soy, corn, eggs and see if you see improvement in their constipation. Be very strict for 3-6 months while you give your child's gut a chance to heal, then add the foods back in, one at a time, seeing if you get a reaction or worsening of constipation or gut pain when you add them back in.

Doctors often tell you that diet isn't causing constipation and gut issues. I don't believe that. You wouldn't put diesel fuel in a race car and you shouldn't put toxic, processed food in your digestive system.

Once you have eliminated things from your diet that are causing inflammation, then it is time to add in things that heal the gut. Bone broth, probiotics, aloe, fermented foods and drinks, and supplements are all avenues to work with to heal the damage done to your gut by constipation and by laxatives.

Bone broth is easy to make and inexpensive. If you can afford it, use organic bones and organic veggie scraps. You can make your own bone broth, which is rich in gut healing collagen and gelatin or you can buy bone broth if you don't have the time to make it.

This is not the stock you buy in a carton. You need a high-quality broth. Bone broth is rich in minerals such as calcium, magnesium, silicon, phosphorus, and sulfur in forms that are easily used by your body. Bone broth also contains glucosamine and chondroitin, which are most often talked about as expensive supplements that help with arthritic joints. Bone Broth also has amino acids which reduce inflammation. Using bone broth in soups, to cook rice or quinoa or a couple of cups in your spaghetti sauce is also an excellent way to get collagen, gelatin and minerals in your gut. These are helpful in strengthening the lining of your intestines.

Bone broth is also very easily digested so you get the benefit of the nutrients in it. This is very important because you need the nutrients to heal but if your gut is inflamed, it is hard to digest nutrient-rich foods.

You can also buy collagen and gelatin, which has amino acids in it, to help build the tissue in the intestines and colon. Collagen is the main structural protein that forms the connective tissue in the gut and helps to seal the lining of the intestines. If you have leaky gut, collagen is really important.

A lack of good gut bacteria or an overabundance of damaging gut bacteria can cause problems in your gut. My son had IV antibiotics at 16 months when he contracted Salmonella. He had constipation issues from birth due to having Megacolon but the IV antibiotics, while they saved his life and were very necessary, also worsened his constipation issues.

If you had antibiotics during pregnancy or delivery or your child had antibiotics at birth or due to illness, then working to repopulating the gut with high-quality bacteria is critical to healing the gut and helping with constipation.

You need good bacteria to digest your food. Even if your child has never been exposed to antibiotics, much of our food, especially meat and dairy products, have antibiotics in them, so just about everyone needs to work on repopulating their gut bacteria.

Traditionally, much of our food would have been fermented. This would have preserved the food but also brought a variety of good bacteria into our gut. Fermented foods and drinks are still one of the best and least expensive ways to re-populate your gut. Many foods that were fermented 100 years ago, like pickles or sauerkraut, are now made with chemical preservatives. It is very easy to make your own fermented foods. Or you can buy naturally fermented foods if you don't want to make them at home.
But lacto-fermented foods are very simple to make and much less expensive. All you need is your vegetable that you are going to ferment, Celtic Sea Salt, filtered water and a canning jar.

Kombucha is a soda-like drink that is full of great bacteria. You can also make your own Kombucha. If you have a child struggling with constipation, this is a fun family project and because it is a soda-like drink, it is often well accepted by picky kids who aren't willing to try other fermented foods. Kimchi and Miso are also wonderful fermented options.

A super easy way to get some good bacteria is using a fermented apple cider vinegar like Bragg's Apple Cider Vinegar or any other vinegar that has the "mother" in it. You can use the vinegar in salad dressings or in dips. I use it in my bone broth to get more minerals out of the bones, in spaghetti sauces and anywhere I can sneak in a teaspoon or tablespoon.

Another simple and fun way to repopulate gut bacteria is to go outside and breathe! We spend so much time indoors in air-conditioned homes and air-conditioned cars and air conditioned office buildings and schools that we rarely breathe unfiltered outdoor air.

Getting outdoors and breathing in air from lots of different places including oceans, lakes, forests, mountains, and deserts, all have different bacteria in the air and will improve the variety of the bacteria in your gut. My husband has Crohn's disease and when he starts to struggle a bit, one of the first things we do is book a trip to the beach or go camping, where he can get the benefit of different bacteria in the air. It always seems to give him a boost.

Antibacterial soap and hand sanitizer kill off good bacteria along with the bad. Use a soap like Dr. Bronner's or another soap with minimal ingredients, essential oils for scents and no added antibacterials.

One of the things that have been most helpful to my family in healing my son and husband's guts is the supplement <u>Restore</u>. It works by sealing the tight junctions in the gut and restoring cell to cell communication in the intestinal lining.

My husband has been taking Restore for close to 7 years and my son for 6. It has been life-changing and improving for them both. They take 1 tsp 3X a day. When my son was in a critical place, we dosed him with 3-5 drops each hour, when he was awake.

Restore can initially increase constipation. This sounds super scary when you're already dealing with constipation but it is a very temporary issue and can be counteracted with magnesium and increasing your child's hydration. Many people do not see any increase of constipation but it might happen so I wanted to give you a heads up.

For my son, who has struggled with constipation his entire life, it has been the key to healing. He currently only takes Restore. He no longer needs laxatives or even magnesium, and as his gut has healed, his other issues caused by Miralax such as tics, OCD etc have also stopped.

Restore is almost tasteless so a wonderful choice for children who have aversions or sensory issues. Restore is about as close to tasteless as you can get. I think before you get super worried that your kid won't take it, just try giving the drops by mouth. And I know, I have a kid that we have to practically sit on to give medicine to, but this is really no big deal and he has taken this fine from the beginning. Now I put his dose in a small shot glass and he drinks it right down. That seems to be easier for us than pouring into a spoon and not losing any on the way to his mouth.

You can also get a pump for your bottle of Restore that squirts out 1 tsp. The pump seems to make our bottle of Restore last longer which keeps costs down. My son also takes it from a spoon for me easily. We also keep a small bottle in my purse and he will take drops from the bottle when we aren't home. We just squirt a little in his mouth. If it is really impossible to get your child to take it by mouth, then you can put it in a drink but it is much harder to make sure they get it all when you are talking about 3 drops to 1 tsp.

Aloe is also wonderful for healing the gut and can help with constipation as well. Just like you put Aloe on a burn or cut on your skin and it helps heal it, taking it internally also soothes and heals damage in your intestines. George's Aloe is a good option for children because they remove the chemical antagonists and some of the mildly toxic ingredients that cause aloe to taste bitter. George's Aloe is virtually tasteless. You can mix it with juice or in soft foods to get your child to drink it.

L-glutamine is an amino acid and a building block of protein cells in your body and is wonderful for healing leaky gut. Typical dosing is 2-5 grams twice daily, taken with a meal. L-glutamine is very helpful if your child has been diagnosed with IBS, Crohn's, Ulcerative Colitis or Diverticulitis. L-Glutamine reduces inflammation in the gut too. My husband has had good success with taking L-glutamine and many of the members of my group have used L-Glutamine with their children and have reported back that they are very happy with the results. Bone broth, grass-fed beef, asparagus, wild caught salmon, turkey and spirulina are all good sources of L-glutamine which you can add to your child's diet.

It can be challenging to make the changes that are needed to heal your child's gut but seeing them grow and flourish makes it all worth it. My son didn't grow well for years when he was struggling with constipation and on Miralax, but as we've healed his gut, he has shot up and is growing like a weed. His anxiety is gone, he's meeting all of his milestones and is healthier than ever.

I hope that this book helps you to find a regiment that helps your child so that he or she can flourish, constipation free.

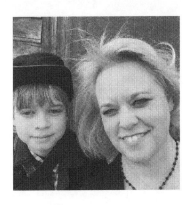

About the Author

Wendy is an author, advocate, wife, and mother who has had extensive personal experience dealing with constipation and gastrointestinal issues because her husband has Crohn's and her youngest son has Celiac and Megacolon. She is not a doctor or a medical professional. She is a woman who was determined to help her family.

Wendy's son was put on Miralax at age 4 for his chronic constipation. He suffered horrible side effects, including tics, anxiety, panic attacks, night terrors, mouth sores, slurred speech and delayed development. After seeing her son struggle with multiple health and neurological issues from Miralax, she decided that there had to be a better way than toxic medicines.

Under the care of an amazing Integrative Medicine doctor, she worked to find the root cause of her son's health issues.

Seeing the huge improvements in her son's health with the changes she made, she decided to share what she had learned with other families who were struggling with constipation and gut issues. Wendy has had the privilege to help thousands of families like hers to end their struggles with chronic constipation and undo the damage that the constipation caused.

Made in the USA
Middletown, DE
09 July 2021